DATE DUE

Color Atlas of

ORAL PATHOLOGY

Color Atlas of

ORAL PATHOLOGY

John W. Eveson

BSc BDS PhD

FDSRCS FDSRCPS FRCPATH

Reader in Oral Medicine and Pathology
Centre for the Study of Oral Diseases
Bristol Dental Hospital and School
Bristol, UK

Crispian Scully

MD PhD MDS FDSRCPS

FFDRCSI FDSRCS FRCPATH

Dean, Eastman Dental Institute for
Oral Healthcare Sciences
University of London
London, UK

M Mosby-Wolfe

London Baltimore Bogotá Boston Buenos Aires Caracas Carlsbad, CA Chicago Madrid Mexico City Milan Naples, FL New York Philadelphia St. Louis Sydney Tokyo Toronto Wiesbaden

Copyright © 1995 Times Mirror International Publishers Limited.

Published in 1995 by Mosby-Wolfe, an imprint of Times Mirror International Publishers Limited.

Printed by Grafos S. A. Arte sobre papel, Barcelona, Spain.

ISBN 0 7234 21129

For full details of all Times Mirror International Publishers Limited titles, please write to Times Mirror International Publishers Limited, Lynton House, 7–12 Tavistock Square, London WC1H 9LB, England.

A CIP catalogue record for this book is available from the British Library.

Library of Congress Cataloging-in-Publication Data applied for.

Project Manager: Alison Taylor

Developmental Editor: Lucy Hamilton

Designer: Judith Gauge

Cover Design: Ian Spick

Illustration: Paul Phillips

Production: Mike Heath

Index: Nina Boyd

Publisher: Geoff Greenwood

To our
long-suffering wives,
Susan and Zoe,
for their unfailing support.

CONTENTS

PREFACE

This manual is intended to be a basic guide to identifying the histological features of the more common or important oral diseases. It makes no pretence to be a comprehensive or balanced account of oral pathology. As it is essentially a practical guide which should be particularly useful to those with limited access to histopathological material, the more theoretical and controversial aspects of the subject are not discussed and references are reduced to a bare minimum. The manual should be of value to dental undergraduates in the oral disease part of the course, dental postgraduates studying for Fellowship examinations and for clinicians specialising in other disciplines such as general histopathology, dermatology and ear, nose and throat surgery.

We are most grateful to Mrs Kathleen Parkes and Mrs Sally Parker for undertaking the onerous task of typing and word processing the text.

John W. Eveson
Crispian Scully

FURTHER READING

Barrett A. W. and Scully C. *Human Oral Mucosal Melanocytes: A Review* (1994). J. Oral Pathol. 23: 97–103.

Berkowitz B. K. B., Holland G. R. and Moxham B. J. *A Colour Atlas and Text of Oral Anatomy, Histology and Embryology*. Wolfe, London, 1992.

Brown R. S., Bottomley W. K., Puente E. and Lavigne G. L. *A Retrospective Evaluation of 193 Patients with Oral Lichen Planus* (1993). J. Oral Pathol. Med. 22: 69–72.

Buchner A., Leider A. S. and Merrell P. W. *Melanocytic Nevi of the Oral Mucosa: A Clinicopathologic Study of 130 Cases from Northern California* (1990). J. Oral Pathol. Med. 19: 197–201.

Cawson R. A. *Essentials of Dental Surgery and Pathology*. 5th Edition. Churchill Livingstone, Edinburgh, 1991.

Cawson R. A., Binnie W. H. and Eveson J. W. *Color Atlas of Oral Disease: Clinical and Pathologic Correlations*. 2nd Edition. Wolfe, London, 1994.

Chou L., Ficarra G. and Hansen L.S. *Hyaline Ring Granuloma: A Distinct Oral Entity* (1990). Oral Surg. Oral Med. Oral Pathol. 70: 318–324.

Eisen D. and Voorhees J. J. *Oral Melanoma and Other Pigmented Lesions of the Oral Cavity* (1991). J. Am. Acad. Dermatol. 24: 527–537.

Enzinger F. M. and Weiss S. W. *Soft Tissue Tumors*. 2nd Edition. Mosby, St Louis, 1988.

Eufinger H., Machtens E., and Akuamoa-Boateng E. *Oral Manifestations of Wegener's Granulomatosis. Review of the Literature and Report of a Case* (1992). Int. J. Oral Maxillofac. Surg. 21: 50–53.

Frank R. M. *Structural Events in the Caries Process in Enamel, Cementum, and Dentin* (1990). J. Dent. Res. 69: 559–565.

Jones J. H. and Mason D. K. *Oral Manifestations of Systemic Disease*. 2nd Edition. Balliere Tindall, London, 1990.

Lozada-Nur F., Gorsky M. and Silverman S. *Oral Erythema Multiforme: Clinical Observations and Treatment of 95 Patients* (1989). Oral Surg. Oral Med. Oral Pathol. 67: 36–40.

Pindborg J. J. *Pathology of the Dental Hard Tissues*. Munksgaard, Copenhagen, 1970.

Scully C., Flint S. and Porter S. R. *An Atlas of Stomatology: Oral Diseases and Manifestations of Systemic Disease*. 2nd Edition. Martin Dunitz, London, 1995.

Scully C. *The Mouth and Perioral Tissues in Health and Disease*. Heinemann, Oxford, 1989.

Scully C. and Samaranayake L. P. *Clinical Virology in Oral Medicine and Dentistry*. Cambridge University Press, Cambridge, 1992.

Seifert G. *WHO International Histological Classification of Tumours. Histological Typing of Salivary Gland Tumours*. Springer-Verlag, Berlin, 1991.

Seifert G., Miehlke A., Haubrich J. and Chilla R. *Diseases of the Salivary Glands*. Georg Thieme Verlag, Stuttgart, 1986.

Shear M. *Cysts of the Oral Region*. 2nd Edition. Wright, Bristol, 1983.

Shear M. *Developmental Odontogenic Cysts. An Update* (1994). J. Oral Pathol. Med. 23: 1–11.

Slootweg P. J. and Muller H. *Differential Diagnosis of Fibro-osseous Jaw Lesions. A Histological Investigation on 30 Cases* (1990). J. Craniomaxillofac. Surg. 18: 210–214.

Soames J. V. and Southam J. C. *Oral Pathology*. 2nd Edition. Oxford Medical Publications, Oxford, 1993.

Ten Cate A. R. *Oral Histology. Development, Structure and Function*. 4th Edition. Mosby, St Louis, 1994.

Thomas D. W. and Shepherd J. P. *Paget's Disease of Bone: Current Concepts in Pathogenesis and Treatment* (1994). J. Oral Pathol. Med. 23: 12–16.

Williams A. J. K., Wray D. and Ferguson A. *The Clinical Entity of Orofacial Crohn's Disease* (1991). Q. J. Med. 79: 451–458.

Williams D. M. *Vesiculo-bullous Mucocutaneous Disease: Benign Mucous Membrane and Bullous Pemphigoid* (1990). J. Oral Pathol. Med. 19: 16–23.

Williams D. M. *Vesiculobullous Mucocutaneous Disease: Pemphigus Vulgaris* (1990). J. Oral Pathol. Med. 18: 544–553.

Williams D. M., Hughes F. J., Odell E. W. and Farthing P. M. *Pathology of Periodontal Disease*. Oxford University Press, Oxford, 1992.

1.
NORMAL ANATOMY AND DEVELOPMENT

EMBRYOLOGY OF TEETH

Tooth formation normally starts at six to eight weeks of foetal development. The sagittal section of a foetal head illustrates some of the earliest stages (**1.1**). Initially, there is a downgrowth of a primary epithelial band (**1.2**) in the lateral region of the maxillary and mandibular processes. This splits into an outer **vestibular lamina,** which will eventually separate the lip from the alveolus, and an inner **dental lamina,** in which areas of condensation (enamel organs) appear which eventually form the teeth.

At a later stage of development (**1.3**), the mandible has started to form a gutter of bone. Meckel's cartilage is found on the medial aspect of the bone and is eventually replaced by it. Meckel's cartilage is therefore merely a supporting structure rather than a definitive embryological precursor. The coarse and woven bone of the mandible is formed by metaplasia of the surrounding fibrous tissue — a type of intramembranous ossification. The bone is rich in osteoblasts, lacks reversal lines, and has no evidence of lamination or osteone (Haversian canal) formation at this stage.

The dental lamina starts to differentiate as a bud-like process that grows down into the embryonic jaw (**1.3**). The lower part indents and becomes cap shaped and at the same time there is condensation of the adjacent connective tissue (**1.4**). This is ectomesenchyme, derived from the neural crest, which forms the embryonic pulp and the fibrous follicle. A layer of columnar cells appears in the lower part of the enamel organ, the **internal enamel epithelium**, which gives rise to the ameloblasts. The outermost layer of cells is more cuboidal and forms the **external enamel epithelium.** The two enamel epithelia are in continuity at the point which eventually becomes the cervical loop. This structure forms Hertwig's sheath which outlines the form of the root. Between the two enamel epithelia is a syncytium-like arrangement of cells called the **stellate reticulum** which appears to have a mainly supporting function.

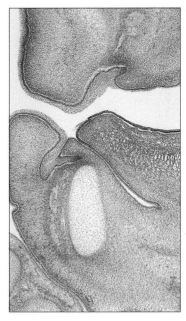

1.1 Primary epithelial band.

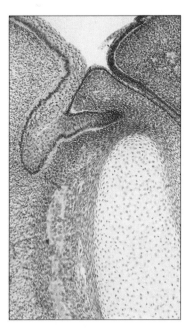

1.2 Primary epithelial band.

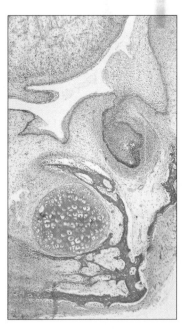

1.3 Bud stage.

In the internal enamel epithelium there is usually a small condensation of cells at the maximum concavity which is called the **enamel knot**. There is also a condensation of flattened cells between the internal enamel epithelium and the stellate reticulum called the **stratum intermedium** which becomes more conspicuous later in development.

1.5 shows an **enamel organ** of a deciduous tooth at the so-called bell stage. Although this is still attached to the surface epithelium by the dental lamina, the latter eventually breaks down, often leaving multiple epithelial rests which become the **rests or glands of Serres**. Successional permanent teeth appear as outgrowths from the enamel organ close to its attachment to the dental lamina. A dense condensation of mesenchyme forms below and around the enamel epithelium and cells in the internal enamel epithelium differentiate into **ameloblasts**. The stellate reticulum is now much more conspicuous. The bone of the mandible is still coarse and woven. The inferior alveolar artery and the mandibular nerve begin to form, and remnants of Meckel's cartilage persist on the medial aspect.

1.6 is a higher power view of the **enamel organ** before hard-tissue formation begins. The internal enamel epithelium is in continuity with the external enamel epithelium at the cervical loop and surrounds the **dental pulp**. This is a very richly cellular mesenchyme, the inner layer of which eventually differentiates into odontoblasts and forms **dentine**. A layer of ameloblasts is starting to differentiate from the internal enamel epithelium. The external enamel epithelium is surrounded by a condensation of connective tissue which will form the **dental follicle**.

1.7 shows a fully formed enamel organ. There is a distinct tooth-like shape with two cusps, one of which shows dentine and enamel matrix formation. The cervical loop is clearly seen where the two enamel epithelia fuse together to form Hertwig's sheath.

The differentiation of ameloblasts and the stratum intermedium (which is only over the part of the internal enamel epithelium that forms enamel) can be seen at higher power (**1.8**). The ameloblasts are palisaded with nuclei polarised away from the basement membrane and are producing a densely purple-staining enamel matrix (haematoxylin and eosin). The immature pulp is vascular and richly cellular. Odontoblasts have differentiated at the pulpo-dentinal junction and have started to deposit dentine. These have elongated processes which are enclosed in tubules (**dentinal tubules**). Thus, enamel is being deposited by the ameloblasts which are migrating in

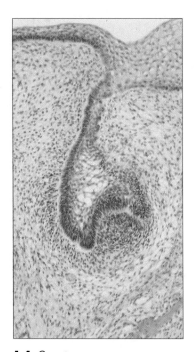

1.4 Cap stage.

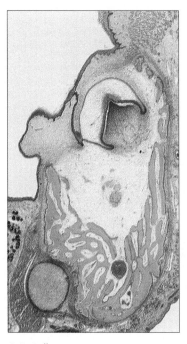

1.5 Bell stage.

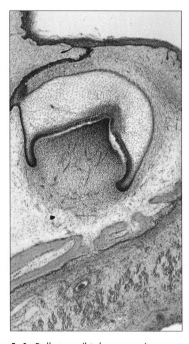

1.6 Bell stage (higher power).

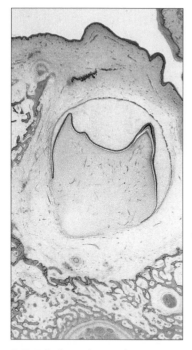

1.7 Fully formed enamel organ.

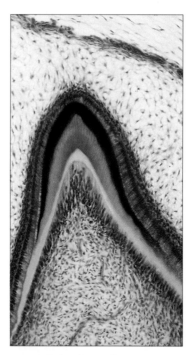

1.8 Early hard-tissue formation at cusp tip.

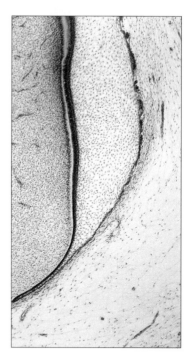

1.9 Cervical loop becoming Hertwig's sheath.

a coronal direction, and odontoblasts which are depositing dentine, are moving in a cervical direction.

Once tooth formation is complete, the stellate reticulum is obliterated and the external enamel epithelium fuses with the internal enamel epithelium to form the **reduced enamel epithelium**.

Hertwig's sheath proliferates apically mapping out the form of the tooth root (**1.9**). This eventually breaks down allowing contact between the surface of the root and the surrounding fibrous tissue which becomes the periodontal ligament (**1.10**). The remnants of Hertwig's sheath form a persistent meshwork

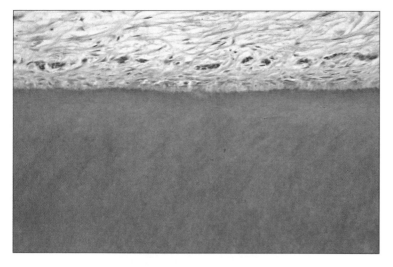

1.10 Breakdown of Hertwig's sheath.

of epithelial cells surrounding the root known as the **cell rests of Malassez** (1.11). The function (if any) of the cell rests of Malassez is unknown but they certainly play a role in the development of some odontogenic cysts, particularly those associated with periapical inflammation.

1.12 shows the alveolar mucosa of a newborn child with numerous odontogenic cell rests which have been derived from the dental lamina (Serres rests). These are often a striking feature of tissue from a foetus or infant and frequently undergo cystic change. Indeed, they sometimes form visible cysts on the infant's alveolus known as Epstein's pearls or Bohn's nodules. Usually these cysts involve spontaneously or fuse with the surface, rupture and disappear. They rarely cause any significant clinical problems. Serres rests may also be important in the formation of some odontogenic tumours and cysts, particularly keratocysts.

Coarse lamellar bone is found on the lamina dura side of the alveolus with prominent incremental lines giving rise to the name of **bundle bone** (**1.13**). Refractile collagen fibres (Sharpey's fibres) penetrate the area of bone adjacent to the periodontal ligament. The periodontal ligament is attached to the cementum and bone. Cementum is a bone-like material which covers the outer surface of the root. The first formed cementum covers the whole root surface.

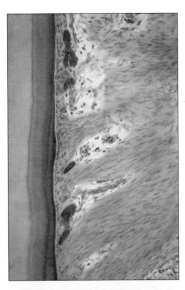

1.11 Cell rests of Malassez in periodontal ligament.

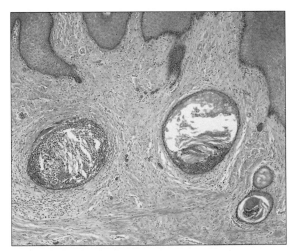

1.12 Serres rests undergoing cystic degeneration.

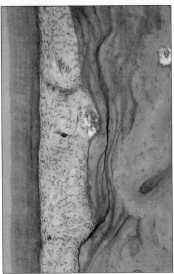

1.13 Acellular cementum, periodontal ligament and bundle bone of alveolus.

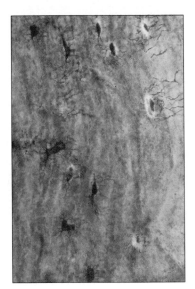

1.14 Cellular cementum. Picrothionin stain.

This early material is acellular and contains incremental lines (lines of Salter). Cellular cementum is incrementally deposited mainly over the apical third of the root and increases in quantity with age. Cellular cementum possesses cementocytes in lacunae. These are the equivalent of osteocytes in bone and are formative cells incarcerated in calcified tissue (**1.14**). The only essential difference between cementum and bone is that cementum is attached to the tooth — otherwise they are biochemically and physically indistinguishable and possess almost identical structure. One structural difference is, however, that the canaliculi of bone osteocytes radiate in all directions, whereas in the cellular cementum they tend to point towards the periodontal ligament from where they gain their nutritional requirements.

NORMAL MUCOSA

The oral mucosa can be divided into the outer epithelial component, which is the equivalent of the epidermis of skin, and the underlying connective tissue. The latter is the equivalent of the cutaneous dermis and can be called the lamina propria or, as now, the corium. The interface between these tissues is the epithelio-mesenchymal junction. This typically undulates due to the presence of rete ridges (**1.15**). The connective tissue bounded by the rete ridges is termed the papillary corium. Below this lies the superficial corium which contains a rather loose network of fine collagen fibres. In the deeper corium, the collagen fibres are coarser and more tightly packed and tend to be aligned parallel to the surface.

The epithelium consists predominantly of keratinocytes with a variety of other cells termed collectively non-keratinocytes. The cells in contact with the basement membrane are cuboidal or columnar in shape and have a relatively high nuclear–cytoplasmic ratio. These form the progenitor layer or stratum germinativum (**1.16**). Although the majority of mitoses occur here, cell division is also occasionally found in the immediate suprabasal layer.

The cells above the basal layer are larger and typically possess prominent intercellular bridges forming the prickle cell layer or stratum spinosum. The long axis of the cells tends to lie parallel to the surface, a feature which becomes more pronounced as the cells differentiate and progressively flatten towards the surface.

When a distinct horny surface layer exists (orthokeratinisation) there is typically a granular cell layer, when the cells contain angular, basophilic keratohyaline granules. In parakeratotic epithelium, an eosinophilic layer of surface keratin with retention of pyknotic nuclei exists. The granular layer is then typically absent.

In non-keratinised epithelium the superficial cells are less flattened and also show less eosinophilia. The most important non-keratinocytes are melanocytes (see section on pigmentation), Langerhan's cells and Merkel cells.

Langerhan's cells appear as clear cells with small dark nuclei in the mid-stratum spinosum on haematoxylin and eosin stained sections. Staining them with alkaline phosphatase and S100 stain, however, shows the cells to be dendritic. They are part of the mononuclear phagocyte system and have an important role in antigen presentation.

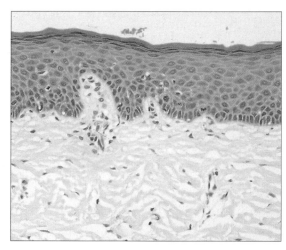

1.15 Oral mucosa — general architecture.

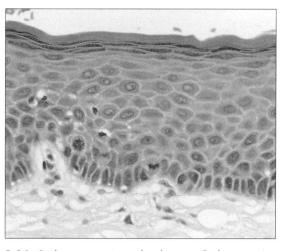

1.16 Oral mucosa — general architecture (higher power).

Merkel cells also appear as clear cells, typically at the tips of the rete ridges in the basal, or immediately suprabasal, layer. These cells have intracellular granules containing catecholamines and are associated with autonomic nerve fibres. Their function is unknown.

REGIONAL VARIATIONS

Tongue and floor of mouth

The ventral lingual mucosa and floor of the mouth are composed of thin, non-keratinised epithelium with short rete ridges (**1.17**). The corium is vascular and has frequent minor sublingual glands (glands of Blandin and Nuhn).

The epithelium of the dorsum of the tongue is thick and covered with papillae, the most numerous of which are the filiform type which are conical with a central connective tissue core. The tongue surface is heavily keratinised and often contains bacterial conglomerates in the superficial layers (**1.18**). The fungiform papillae are much less numerous rounded elevations, which may be keratinised or non-keratinised, and usually contain taste buds in the upper surface. The circumvallate papillae are 10–12 in number and lie in front of the sulcus terminalis. Each circumvallate papilla lies in a deep circular groove. The epithelium lining this groove and the papilla surface contains many taste buds. Minor serous salivary glands (von Ebner's glands) open into the base of the grooves. Several leaf-shaped (foliate)

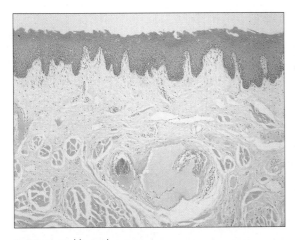

1.17 Ventral lingual mucosa.

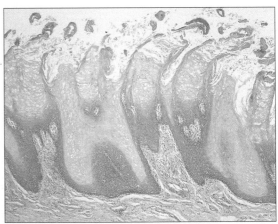

1.18 Dorsal lingual mucosa.

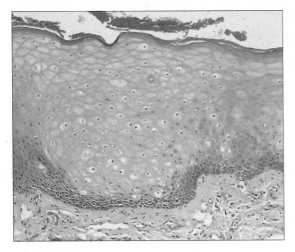

1.19 Buccal mucosa.

1.20 Fordyce spot.

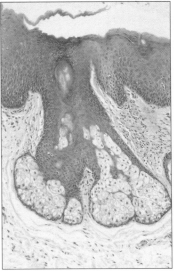

papillae may occur on the lateral border of the tongue immediately in front of the palato-glossal fold. These contain lymphoid tissue in their connective tissue core similar to the rest of Waldeyer's ring. Irritation, inflammation and enlargement of these foliate papillae is common.

Buccal mucosa

The cheeks are lined by thick, non-keratinised epithelium with a relatively flat epithelio-mesenchymal junction and few rete ridges (**1.19**). A white line (linea alba), which is usually parakeratinised, is commonly seen opposite the occlusal line. The buccal mucosa (and upper lip) is a common site for sebaceous glands known as Fordyce spots or granules (**1.20**). These have no associated hair follicles and open onto the surface by a short duct. Fordyce spots tend to increase in number with age but their function is obscure.

Palate

The epithelium of the hard palate is orthokeratinised and usually possesses many long rete ridges (**1.21**). These become less conspicuous towards the midline. The soft palate is lined by thinner, non-keratinised epithelium and overlies numerous, minor mucous salivary glands.

Lips

The labial mucosa is lined by thick, non-keratinised epithelium with short blunt rete ridges (**1.22**). Fordyce spots are common in the upper lip and minor salivary glands are present in the submucosa of both upper and lower lips.

SALIVARY GLANDS

Salivary glands are divided into major and minor glands. The major glands are the parotid, submandibular and sublingual glands. Minor glands are found in the lips, soft palate, buccal mucosa, retromolar pads, sublingually (occasionally extending to the tip of the tongue) and in the pharynx and tonsils.

The parenchyma consists of varying proportions of serous and mucous cells forming acini, and ducts. The serous cells are triangular and have basophilic granular cytoplasm. Mucous cells have pale, vacuolated cytoplasm and the nucleus is typically flattened against the base of the cell.

The parotid gland is purely serous (**1.23**, **1.24**) whereas the submandibular gland is mixed seromucous (with serous cells forming demilunes at the

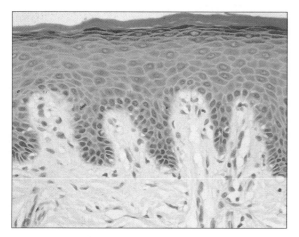

1.21 Palatal mucosa.

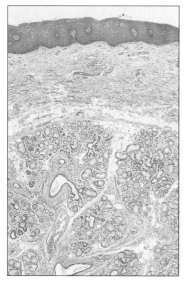

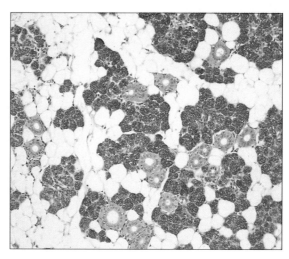

1.22 Labial mucosa with underlying minor salivary glands.

1.23 Parotid gland (low power).

periphery of the acinus) (**1.25, 1.26**). The sublingual gland is also mixed but is predominantly mucous. Most minor glands are mucous (**1.27**) except those in the lips and the minor sublingual glands which are seromucous.

A normal major salivary gland consists of discrete lobes or lobules, separated by fibrous septa. A moderate amount of fat is often present in the lobules, but this is variable and is usually only present in small amounts in the submandibular glands. The striated ducts are fairly numerous and readily seen. The ducts are pink and oncocytic — a term which is used because they are granular as well as pink. The granularity is due to an increase in the number of mitochondria. The ducts appear striated because of the infoldings of the basal aspect of the plasma membrane.

Intralobular ducts pass into the larger septa and join to form interlobular and finally collecting ducts which are usually large, often fairly eosinophilic, and may contain goblet cells. The collecting ducts normally have blood vessels and nerves running with them.

The intercalated ducts and acini have myoepithelial cells on their periphery, under sympathetic and parasympathetic nervous control. The myoepithelial cells cannot be identified in haematoxylin and eosin stained tissue but are readily visualised after immunocytochemical staining for actin or myosin microfilaments.

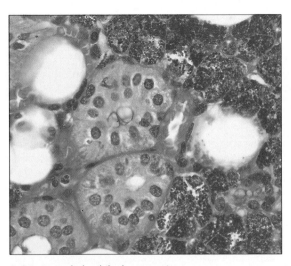

1.24 Parotid gland (higher power).

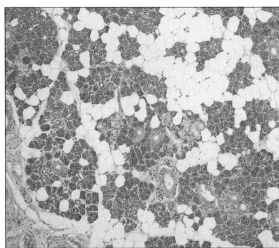

1.25 Submandibular gland (low power).

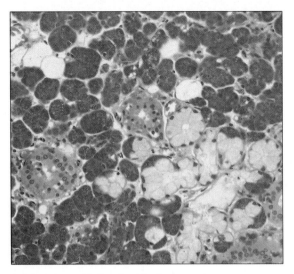

1.26 Submandibular gland (higher power).

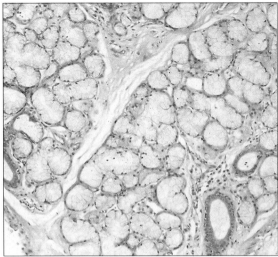

1.27 Mucous glands of the palate.

COMMON VARIATIONS IN SALIVARY HISTOLOGY

The parotid gland always contains considerably more fat than the submandibular gland, the amount of which further increases with age. If sufficient material is examined it is common to find sebaceous tissue in the parotid gland (**1.28**) although sebaceous neoplasms are rare.

Other common findings in the parotid glands are lymph nodes and lymphatic tissue (**1.29**). Salivary lymph nodes frequently contain ducts and sometimes acini (**1.30**). In adults, ducts are usually seen in the intraparotid lymphoid aggregates although in children acini may also appear. These heterotopic ducts are thought to be the progenitors of Warthin's tumours and possibly lymphoepithelial and branchial cysts.

Oncocytosis is the term used to denote the presence of cells which are brightly eosinophilic and densely granular (often throughout the whole cell rather than just the basal part). The nuclei are usually slightly vesicular with an evenly distributed chromatin pattern. Oncocytosis with increasing age is a common finding in ducts and occasionally affects acinar cells (**1.31**).

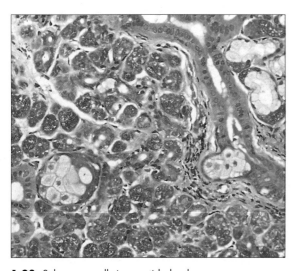

1.28 Sebaceous cells in parotid gland.

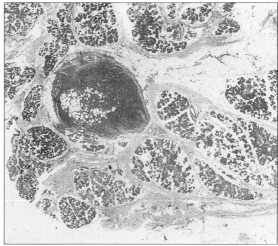

1.29 Intraparotid lymph node.

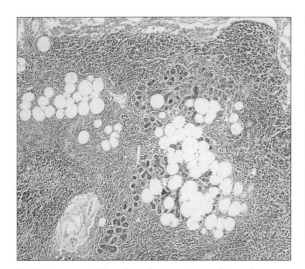

1.30 Intraparotid lymph node containing salivary duct inclusions.

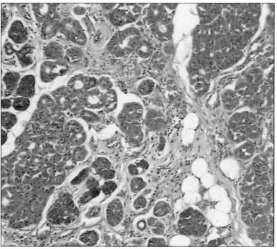

1.31 Oncocytic metaplasia of ducts and acini.

LYMPH NODES

A normal lymph node usually has a discrete capsule below which is a subcapsular sinus and variable numbers of B-cell-derived germinal centres with predominantly T-cell paracortical areas (**1.32**). In a normal lymph node the germinal centres are discrete, usually with a rim of small lymphocytes which can often be delineated from the rest of the lymph node (**1.33**). The germinal centres contain two predominant cell types — centroblasts and centrocytes. Centroblasts are large, pale cells which have a relatively vesicular nucleus and usually one or more prominent nucleoli, often associated with the nuclear membrane. Centrocytes are small cells (although larger than a normal lymphocyte) and have denser cytoplasm and often an indented nucleus (which is why they are sometimes called cleaved cells). Mitotic activity is common within the germinal centre. The other cells seen in germinal centres are large, pale macrophages often containing basophilic, round or angular pieces of cellular debris called tingible bodies (**1.34, 1.35**). Although not an absolute rule, as once thought, the presence of these bodies is a useful indicator of a normal but reactive germinal centre (as it is very uncommon to see tingible-body macrophages in neoplastic follicles).

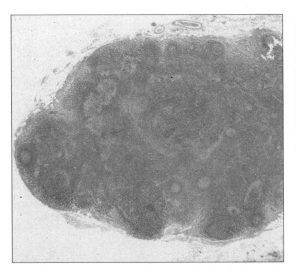

1.32 Lymph node (low power).

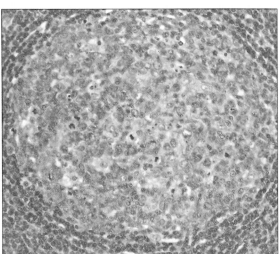

1.33 Germinal centre.

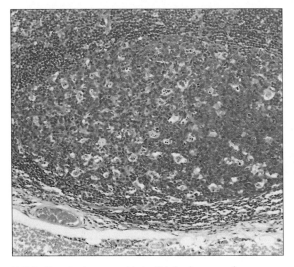

1.34 Germinal centre with tingible-body macrophages.

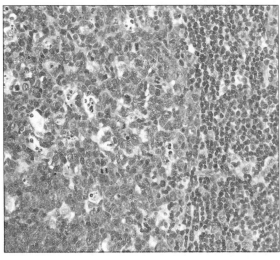

1.35 Germinal centre (higher power).

2.

DEFECTS OF TEETH

DENTINOGENESIS IMPERFECTA (HEREDITARY OPALESCENT DENTINE)

Dentinogenesis imperfecta is usually inherited as an autosomal dominant trait and may be associated with brittle bone disease (osteogenesis imperfecta). It typically affects all the teeth in both dentitions. The enamel is normal in form but is abnormally trans-lucent producing a bluish-brown opalescent appearance. The crown is bulbous and the roots are short with a tendency to pulpal obliteration (**2.1**). There is a defective union between the enamel and dentine so that the enamel readily chips away allowing the underlying defective dentine to wear rapidly. Microscopy shows that the earliest formed (mantle) dentine is usually normal but there is a wide predentine zone with abundant interglobular dentine and vascular inclusions (**2.2**).

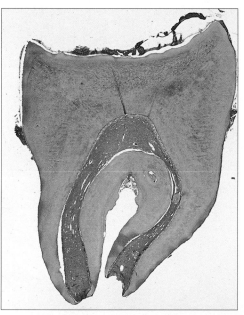

2.1 Dentinogenesis imperfecta.

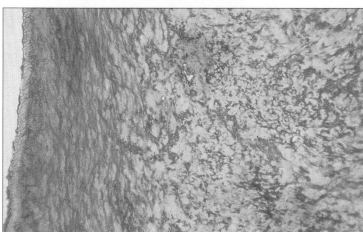

2.2 Dentinogenesis imperfecta with normal mantle denture.

REGIONAL ODONTODYSPLASIA (GHOST TEETH)

This rare disorder is characterised by localised arrest of development of one or several teeth, either deciduous or permanent. The affected teeth fail to erupt and radiographs show ghost-like teeth with crumpled crowns and defective root formation. Microscopy shows hypoplastic, poorly mineralised enamel covered by irregularly calcified, reduced enamel epithelium and follicle. The pulp chamber is wide and there is increased interglobular dentine together with amorphous, grey, collagen-free areas of matrix (**2.3, 2.4**).

RICKETS

Dietary rickets is very uncommon in developed countries where most cases are secondary to renal disease. Affected enamel may be hypoplastic and form pits and grooves. Dentine is poorly mineralised and microscopy shows increased amounts of interglobular dentine and a widened predentine zone (**2.5, 2.6**).

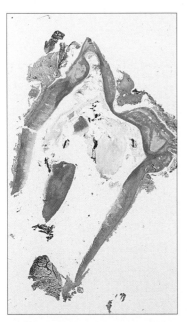

2.3 Regional odontodysplasia.

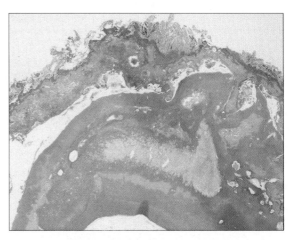

2.4 Regional odontodysplasia.

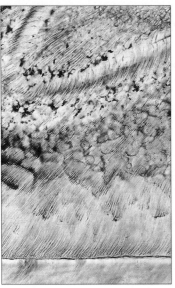

2.5 Renal rickets — undecalcified ground section.

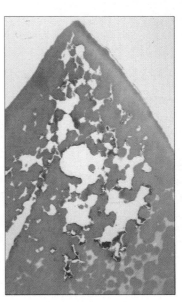

2.6 Renal rickets — decalcified section.

TETRACYCLINE STAINING

Tetracycline is incorporated into calcifying tissues, including developing teeth. It is deposited along incremental lines in both enamel and dentine giving affected teeth a greyish-brown opaque appearance. The staining shows as a bright yellow–green fluorescence when ground sections are visualised under ultraviolet light (**2.7**).

TOOTH RESORPTION

Although deciduous teeth are resorbed physiologically during shedding a variety of pathological processes can give rise to resorption. Tooth resorption can result from trauma, re-implantation, tumours, cysts and inflammatory lesions. Occasionally, resorption (which can be external or internal) is idiopathic. Idiopathic internal resorption is characterised by proliferation of vascular granulation tissue in the pulp and resorption of the adjacent dentine by osteoclast-like (odontoclasts) multinucleated giant cells (**2.8–2.10**). There may be areas of irregular repair with tubular dentine or cementum-like material. Eventually the destruction extends through the enamel and may appear as a pink spot on the surface before pulpal exposure.

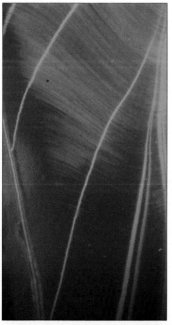

2.7 Tetracycline staining — fluorescent appearance under ultraviolet light.

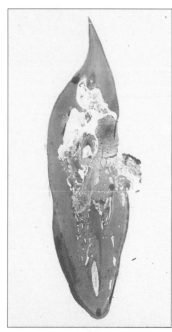

2.8 Internal resorption.

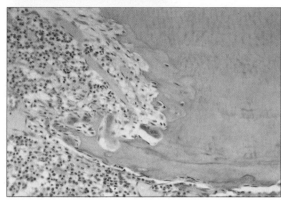

2.9 Internal resorption.

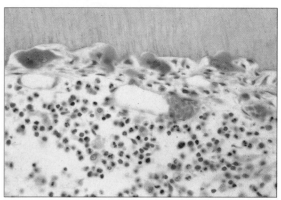

2.10 Osteoclast-like giant cells (odontoclasts) at high power.

3.

CARIES AND PULPITIS

ENAMEL CARIES

The earliest detectable carious lesion is a white spot or opacity in the enamel usually below a contact point or in a pit or fissure. When such lesions are examined in undecalcified ground sections they show a conical area of demineralisation with the apex extending towards the amelodentinal junction (**3.1**). The early lesion can be divided into four zones each of which is produced by demineralisation resulting in pores of variable size and numbers. The advancing edge is a translucent area deep to which is a linear dark zone. The body of the lesion is also somewhat translucent and usually contains enhanced striae of Rhetzius. The surface zone is intact, probably because of reprecipitation of calcium.

The lesion eventually penetrates the full thickness of the enamel and then spreads laterally at the amelodentinal junction to affect a relatively larger area of the underlying dentine (**3.2**). The enamel is thus undermined and weakened and ultimately fractures to leave a cavity (**3.3**). This allows the ingress of bacteria which greatly accelerate the destruction.

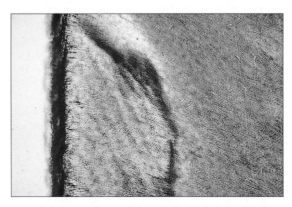

3.1 Undecalcified ground section of early interstitial caries.

DENTINE CARIES

Unlike enamel, dentine can undergo a vital reaction to caries mediated by odontoblasts and other pulpal cells. Bacteria (pioneer organisms) invade and extend down the dentinal tubules (**3.4**). Focal areas become distended with masses of bacteria to form

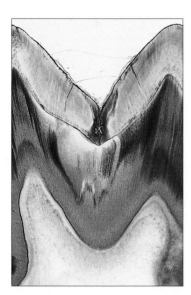

3.2 Undecalcified ground section of fissure caries.

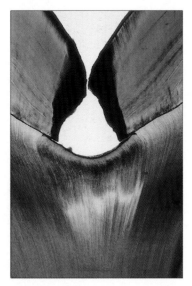

3.3 Undecalcified ground section of advanced fissure caries.

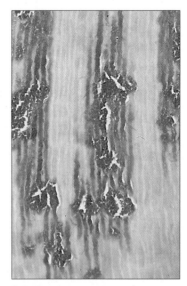

3.4 Pioneer organisms and liquefaction foci in dentine caries.

liquefaction foci which may fuse laterally to form characteristic transverse clefts (**3.5**).

Mineral deposition is found within the dentinal tubules (called intratubular or sometimes, inappropriately, peritubular dentine) at the periphery of the lesion, which can be seen as a translucent zone in undercalcified ground sections. If the carious process is rapid it outstrips the defence mechanisms, the odontoblasts die and the affected area of dentine becomes known as a dead tract. This is usually sealed off at the pulpal end of the tubules by an acellular calcified barrier. Irregular, secondary (reparative) dentine is formed beneath this by the surrounding odontoblasts or cells differentiating from pulpal mesenchymal cells (**3.6**). In rapidly advancing caries these protective barriers are breached and bacteria reach the pulp (**3.7**).

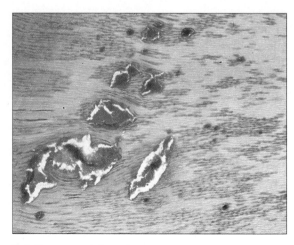

3.5 Transverse clefts in dentine caries.

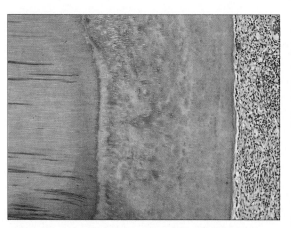

3.6 Pioneer organisms approaching reparative (secondary) dentine.

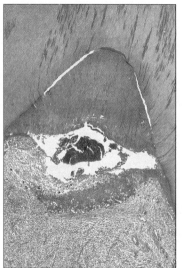

3.7 Caries breaching layer of reparative dentine.

PULPAL DEGENERATION

Although immature pulp contains little collagen, deposition is seen later — especially in the root canals. Older teeth frequently possess diffuse dystrophic calcification which appears as coarse, granular basophilic material.

The pulp illustrated shows irregular pulp stones and diffuse calcifications, but little fibrosis (**3.8**). Pulp stones are areas of dystrophic calcification around small thrombi or nidi of dead tissue (**3.9**). Some pulp stones are concentrically laminated (**3.10**). Pulp stones never cause clinical problems except for blocking access to a root canal for endodontic treatment. The only condition where there are multiple pulp stones is Ehlers–Danlos syndrome.

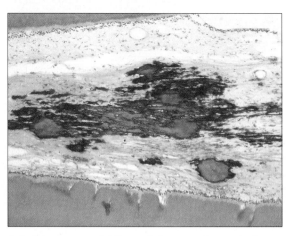

3.8 Pulp stones and diffuse calcifications of root canal.

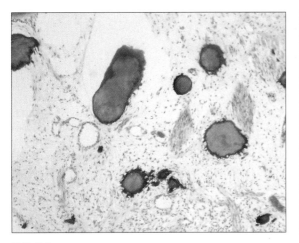

3.9 Pulp stones.

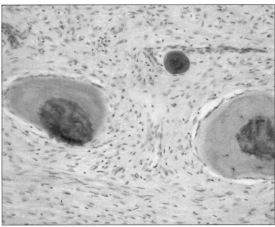

3.10 Concentrically laminated pulp stones.

PULPITIS

The earliest stage of pulpal inflammation is hyperaemia and polymorph emigration in the area of pulp underlying the zone of caries (**3.11**). There is a progressive accumulation of polymorphs which may form a microabscess (**3.12**), particularly in a pulp horn. Usually, however, the inflammation spreads to involve the whole pulp. The inflammatory exudate increases the intrapulpal pressure impairing the pulpal circulation and compressing the vessels in the apical foramina. This rapidly leads to ischaemic pulpal necrosis (**3.13**).

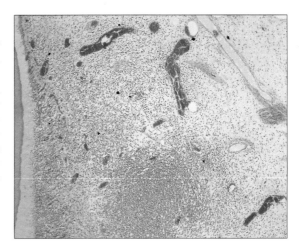

3.11 Pulpal hyperaemia and polymorph infiltration.

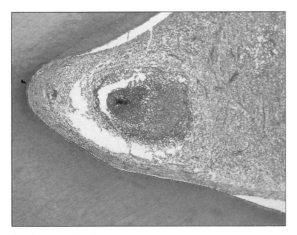

3.12 Coronal pulpal abscess.

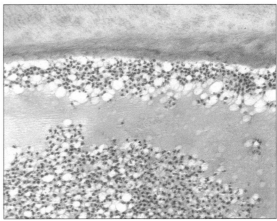

3.13 Pulpal suppuration and necrosis.

CHRONIC PULPITIS

Pulp abscesses occasionally become localised and show chronic inflammation and fibrous repair in the surrounding pulp. Typically, however, there is slow progression of inflammation throughout the pulp with mild vascular dilatation and infiltration of plasma cells and lymphocytes. The pulp may survive for a time even when the overlying dentine has been destroyed — the so-called 'chronic open pulpitis' (**3.14**).

CHRONIC HYPERPLASTIC PULPITIS (PULP POLYP)

Although necrosis is the most common sequel of pulpal inflammation, the pulp occasionally survives even when there has been gross destruction of the overlying enamel and dentine (**3.15**). The remaining pulpal tissue proliferates to form granulation tissue which bulges into the carious cavity as a polyp. The surface eventually becomes epithelialised, the inflammation subsides and the polyp becomes more fibrous.

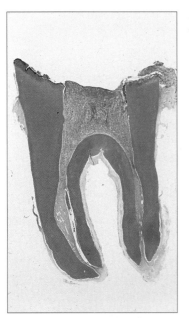

3.14 Chronic open pulpitis.

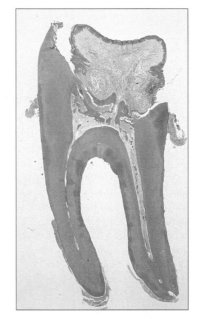

3.15 Chronic hyperplastic pulpitis (pulp polyp).

4.

GINGIVA

GINGIVAL FIBROUS HYPERPLASIA

Gingival fibrous hyperplasia may be either inherited or drug-associated. Hereditary gingival fibromatosis is inherited as an autosomal dominant trait and may be associated with thickening of facial features and hypertrichosis. Microscopy shows grossly increased fibrous tissue which otherwise appears normal apart from superimposed inflammatory changes. There is usually an elongation of the rete ridges of the overlying epithelium (**4.1**). The features are identical in drug-associated gingival hyperplasia.

CHRONIC MARGINAL GINGIVITIS

Chronic marginal gingivitis is characterised microscopically by mild vascular hyperaemia and dense chronic inflammatory infiltrate (**4.2**). The crevicular epithelium may be ulcerated or hyperplastic with irregular anastomosing prolongations into the underlying connective tissue (**4.3**). There is gross intercellular oedema and infiltration of the epithelium by polymorphs. Dense aggregates of plasma cells and lymphocytes, often with granular basophilic extracellular immunoglobulin, are found in the connective tissue (**4.4**). Russell bodies, which consist of precipitated immunoglobulin within plasma cells, may also be plentiful.

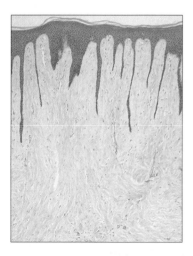

4.1 Fibrous gingival hyperplasia.

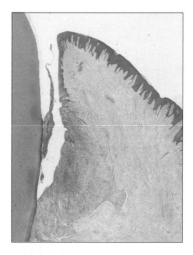

4.2 Chronic marginal gingivitis (low power).

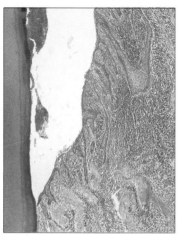

4.3 Chronic marginal gingivitis. Higher power of crevicular epithelium.

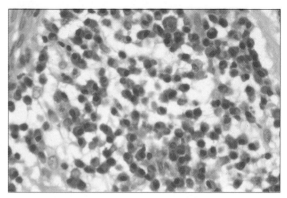

4.4 Higher power of dense plasma cell infiltrate in chronic gingivitis.

WEGENER'S GRANULOMATOSIS

This condition is characterised by necrotising vasculitis, with multinucleated giant cells, typically affecting the nasopharynx and lungs. An uncommon, but very distinctive clinical manifestation is a proliferative gingivitis.

The gingival swellings start interdentally and spread to the marginal gingiva. These have a purplish, mottled appearance that resembles an over-ripe strawberry. Microscopy shows inflammation and areas of recent and old haemorrhage (**4.5**). There is a mixed acute and chronic inflammatory infiltrate, focal aggregates of eosinophils and neutrophils may produce microabscesses (**4.6**). There may be scattered multinucleated giant cells but the vasculitis typical of Wegener's granulomatosis in other sites is not usually seen in gingival biopsies. The overlying epithelium usually shows extensive (pseudoepitheliomatous) hyperplasia.

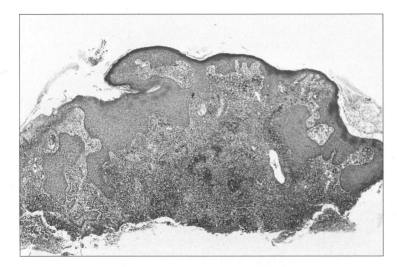

4.5 Wegener's granulomatosis of gingiva.

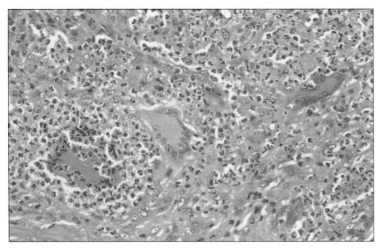

4.6 Wegener's granulomatosis showing polymorph microabscesses and multinucleated giant cells.

5.

CYSTS

PERIAPICAL GRANULOMA AND RADICULAR CYST FORMATION

After the death of the pulp, any microorganisms present are usually located in the root canal or the delta region of the apical area of the tooth (where there are multiple root canals). This induces a chronic inflammatory response at the apex of the tooth. There is a gradually increasing mass of chronic inflammatory cells, predominantly plasma cells and lymphocytes, with variable amounts of fibrosis. This is accommodated within the bone by peripheral resorption of the alveolar bone by osteoclasts to form

a periapical granuloma. The same stimulus that causes the chronic inflammatory response around the apex stimulates the cell rests of Malassez to proliferate, and epithelium starts to permeate the granuloma (**5.1**). The granuloma consists predominantly of chronic inflammatory cells although there is often infiltration of the epithelium by polymorphs. The epithelium shows intercellular oedema which causes breakdown of the epithelial islands and subsequent microcyst formation (**5.2**). The microcysts eventually coalesce to form a central cystic cavity (**5.3**).

5.4 shows a later stage of the process. Central breakdown has ensued and, in some areas of the peri-

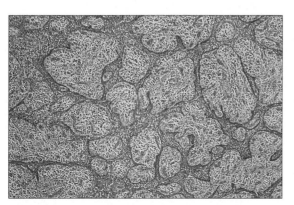

5.1 Epithelial proliferation in periapical granuloma.

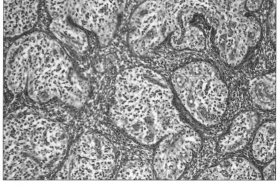

5.2 Epithelial proliferation in periapical granuloma (higher power).

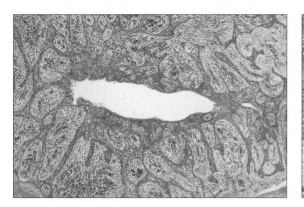

5.3 Early cyst formation in periapical granuloma.

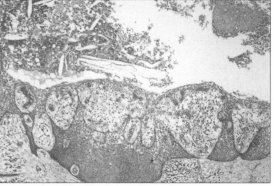

5.4 Hyperplastic epithelium lining radicular cyst.

apical granuloma, arcades of proliferating epithelium can be seen lining the cyst cavity. There is a great deal of blood with haemosiderin and cholesterol clefts in the centre of the cyst and within the fibrous wall (**5.5**). As the inflammation subsides the cyst becomes separated from the inflammatory products in the pulp and becomes lined by stratified squamous epithelium of variable thickness (**5.6**). The mature dental cyst is lined by attenuated stratified squamous epithelium (usually with little inflammation in the fibrous wall although scattered lymphocytes, plasma cells and haemosiderin-containing macrophages may be present (**5.7**)). Sometimes, foamy macrophages (which contain ingested fat) are present within the cyst wall and occasionally they are numerous (**5.8, 5.9**). Mucous metaplasia may arise in radicular cysts (as well as in dentigerous cysts) (**5.10**) and foci of dystrophic calcification appear.

Hyaline (Rushton) bodies can be seen in odontogenic cysts, typically radicular cysts, and occasionally in keratocysts or dentigerous cysts. Some hyaline bodies have a clear, crystalline outline, a hair-pin shape and a tendency to fracture (**5.11**). Other hyaline bodies show a central granular area. Their origin is controversial. It was once thought that they were derived from products of the prominent vessels seen in inflamed radicular cyst linings, but it is now generally accepted that they are a secretory product of the epithelial cells.

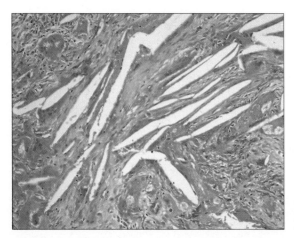

5.5 Cholesterol clefts and haemosiderin deposition in radicular cyst.

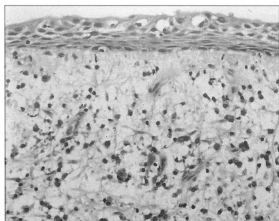

5.6 Wall of radicular cyst.

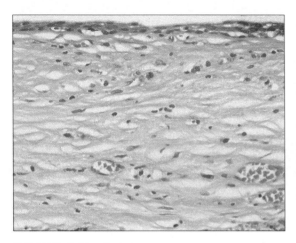

5.7 Wall of old radicular cyst.

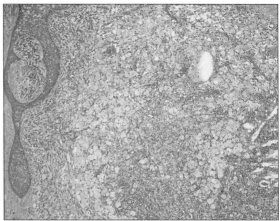

5.8 Foamy macrophages in periapical granuloma.

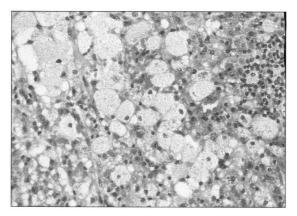

5.9 Foamy macrophages in periapical granuloma (higher power).

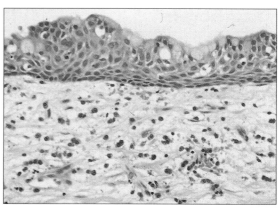

5.10 Mucous metaplasia in radicular cyst.

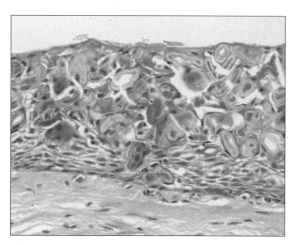

5.11 Hyaline bodies in radicular cyst.

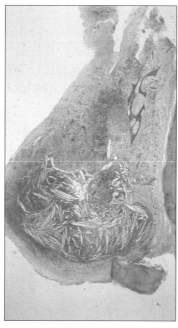

5.12 Paradental cyst.

PARADENTAL CYSTS

Paradental cysts usually arise on the distobuccal aspect of partially erupted lower third molars, in teeth which have associated pericoronitis. Occasionally, a small enamel spur extends between the roots of the tooth and this has been postulated to stimulate cyst formation. The cyst is histologically identical to other periapical or lateral radicular cysts. It is lined by stratified squamous epithelium of variable thickness, is often inflamed and (as in this example) shows florid cholesterol cleft formation and areas of dystrophic calcification (**5.12**). Therefore, the paradental cyst can only be distinguished from any other type of inflammatory odontogenic cyst by clinical and radiological features. The cyst lining probably arises from the cell rests of Malassez.

KERATOCYSTS

Keratocysts probably arise from the dental lamina and, because a tooth is occasionally missing, they are sometimes termed primordial cysts. The large majority of keratocysts arise in the body or ramus of the mandible. They typically form an area of scalloped and pseudo-loculated radiolucency and tend not to expand laterally until they have reached a considerable size.

A non-inflamed keratocyst has a very thin, fibrous wall (**5.13**), which macroscopically looks rather like a collapsed balloon. Typically, it has a thin epithelial lining which is about five to eight cells thick and a corrugated surface (**5.14**). The basal cell layer is palisaded, with a tendency for the nuclei to be polarised away from the basement membrane, rather as in ameloblasts (**5.15**). A prominent basement membrane zone is usually present between the epithelium and the underlying connective tissue. There is a tendency for the epithelium to separate from the wall. The lining often infolds into the underlying connective tissue or may form separate daughter cysts (**5.16**).

The epithelial lining is usually parakeratotic (sometimes with a very thin surface layer of keratin). Rare orthokeratotic variants usually have less typical morphology and often lack palisaded basal cells.

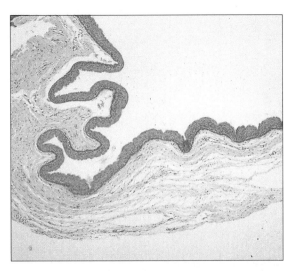

5.13 Keratocyst (low power).

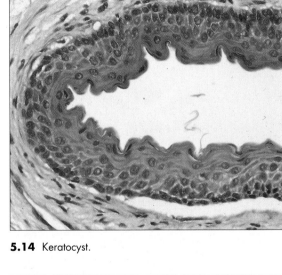

5.14 Keratocyst.

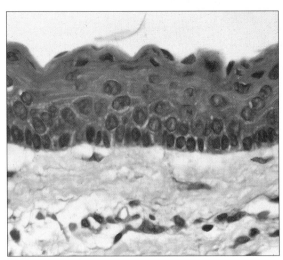

5.15 Keratocyst.

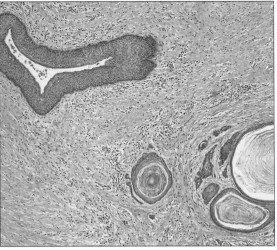

5.16 Satellite (daughter) cysts in keratocyst.

Keratocysts are multiple in about 10% of patients. Multiple keratocysts, together with multiple basal cell naevi and a variety of skeletal defects, constitute the Gorlin–Goltz syndrome. Such patients typically have hypertelorism, and often calcification of the falx cerebri and bifid ribs. Most of the skin tumours, particularly in the early stages, are non-malignant but they may develop into basal cell carcinomas later in the course of the disease.

The relationship between the cyst and bone is seen in **5.17**. Keratocysts tend to spread by mural growth rather than unicystic expansion (which characterises most other cyst development). Keratocysts can reach a very large size before becoming detectable because they spread through the bone interstices in an antero-posterior direction (through cancellous bone) rather than laterally. Another distinguishing feature of keratocysts is that the characteristic features disappear in areas of inflammation (**5.18**) and the lining may look the same as a radicular cyst lining.

Daughter cysts, within the walls of keratocysts, probably arise from the cell rests of Serres and may be numerous (**5.19**). Some may be due to infoldings of the cyst wall rather than separate islands. In any event, they are one of the reasons why keratocysts have a tendency to recur, since daughter cysts remain after surgical removal of the main cyst.

Keratocysts can occasionally appear to be dentigerous upon radiological examination. They may be in either a true dentigerous relationship to the tooth (when the cyst lining is attached at the cervico-enamel junction) or they may be merely envelopmental (when a tooth erupts into, or is surrounded by, an expanding cyst).

Keratocysts can arise on the lateral aspect of the root of a tooth and thus present as a lateral cyst. Most so-called globulo-maxillary cysts are keratocysts or, less frequently, lateral radicular or residual cysts.

5.17 Keratocyst expanding into adjacent bone.

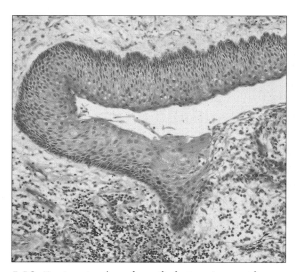

5.18 Keratocyst — loss of specific features in area of inflammation.

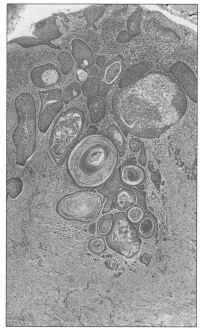

5.19 Florid proliferation in the wall of a keratocyst.

DENTIGEROUS (FOLLICULAR) CYSTS

Dentigerous cysts typically arise in relation to impacted teeth or those which erupt late. They are, therefore, most common in the lower third molar, upper canine and lower second premolar regions. Dentigerous cysts are also called follicular cysts because they arise from fluid accumulation between the reduced enamel epithelium and the enamel of the tooth. The wall of the cyst is therefore formed by the dental follicle while the cyst lining is attached at the cervico-enamel junction. There may be inflammation in the cyst wall around the attachment of the tooth at the cervico-enamel junction (although this is rare in other areas unless the cyst has become secondarily infected). Typically, the cyst wall is sparsely cellular and rich in ground substance rendering fragmented specimens easily confused with a fibromyxoma (**5.20**). The lining of the cyst is variable sometimes being a structured bilayer or simply a flattened stratified squamous epithelium. It is not uncommon to find metaplasia in these cysts, typically mucous metaplasia (**5.21**).

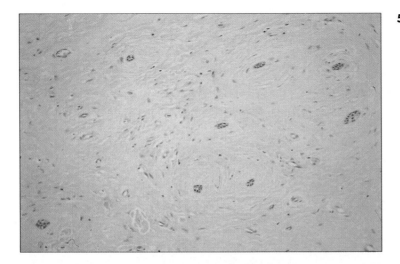

5.20 Dentigerous cyst — fibrous wall.

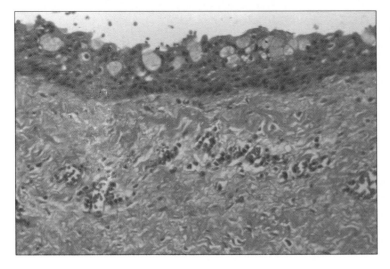

5.21 Mucous metaplasia in wall of dentigerous cyst.

Mucicarmine highlights the extent of the mucous metaplasia seen in some instances (**5.22**). It should be remembered that mucous metaplasia is of no significance and care should be taken not to misdiagnose it as a mucoepidermoid carcinoma (which can also present as a cyst).

Occasionally areas of keratinisation exist (keratinising metaplasia) and aspirates from one of these cysts can sometimes be confused with a keratocyst. There may be proliferation of cell rests of Serres in the cyst wall. Although it is a useful diagnostic feature, the latter can also lead to confusion because it is occasionally extensive and can be confused with an odontogenic tumour (**5.23, 5.24**).

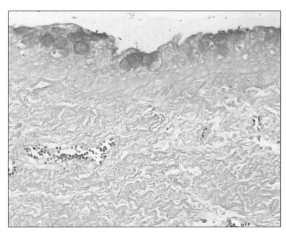

5.22 Mucous metaplasia in wall of dentigerous cyst. Mucicarmine stain.

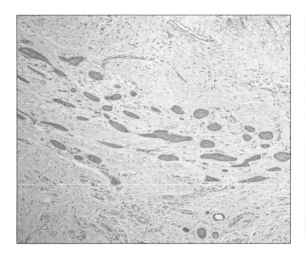

5.23 Proliferation of odontogenic cell rests in wall of dentigerous cyst.

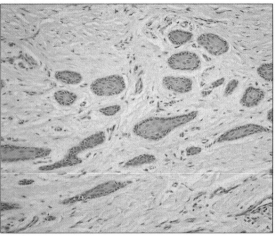

5.24 Proliferation of odontogenic cell rests in wall of dentigerous cyst (higher power).

ERUPTION CYSTS

An eruption cyst is a follicular cyst without overlying bone (the roof of which therefore consists of oral epithelium). Eruption cysts present as bluish swellings overlying the crown of an unerupted deciduous tooth or, occasionally, a permanent molar. They are attached to the cervico-enamel junction. Although eruption cysts are derived from reduced enamel epithelium their lining is usually non-specific. The linings are non-keratinised stratified squamous epithelium which typically show immediately subjacent inflammation (**5.25**).

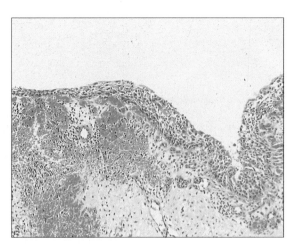

5.25 Eruption cyst.

ANEURYSMAL BONE CYSTS

Aneurysmal bone cysts can arise in either jaw and usually affect young people. They form an expanding cystic lesion which balloons out into the adjacent tissues. Aneurysmal bone cysts are frequently associated with other lesions such as ossifying fibromas or fibrous dysplasia. They often have a substantial multinucleate giant cell element, and may resemble giant cell granulomas of the jaw.

Aneurysmal bone cysts form a sponge-work of vascular spaces, lined by fibrous septa which also show varying degrees of vascularity (**5.26**). Frequently, multinucleated giant cells line the vascular spaces (**5.27**). The stroma contains spindle-shaped cells and a high degree of vascularity, haemorrhage and associated haemosiderin (**5.28**). Osseous metaplasia may be another feature in which woven bone forms within the spindle-cell stroma. This can be florid and may superficially resemble osteosarcoma although there is no cytological atypia. Aneurysmal bone cysts are benign, but recur in a significant number of cases.

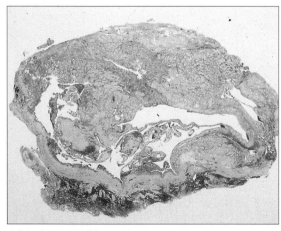

5.26 Aneurysmal bone cyst.

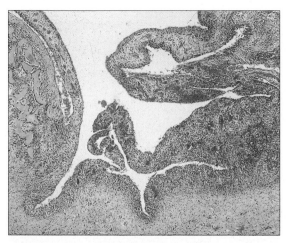

5.27 Aneurysmal bone cyst (higher power).

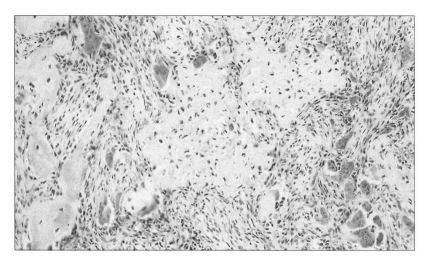

5.28 Osseous metaplasia and multinucleated giant cells in wall of aneurysmal bone cyst.

SIMPLE (TRAUMATIC, HAEMOR-RHAGIC, SOLITARY) BONE CYSTS

Simple bone cysts are typically seen in the lower molar region in patients below the age of 20 years. Often chance findings on radiographs, simple bone cysts usually form a distinct radiolucent area which characteristically arches up between the roots of the teeth. There is often little bony expansion and, when the cyst is opened, it is usually found to be either empty or to contain a small amount of sero-san-guinous fluid. Therefore, the histological specimen is merely the window of bone removed when the cyst was surgically opened and shows a shell of normal bone and variable amounts of fibrous tissue and fibrin (sometimes with occasional multinucleated giant cells) attached to the bony plate (**5.29**). Occasionally an overlap lesion between a simple bone cyst and an aneurysmal bone cyst is seen.

Simple bone cysts usually heal spontaneously after minimal surgical intervention. Indeed, the fact that they are rare in patients over 20 years old suggests that most spontaneously resolve without treatment. It is thought that the cysts arise from trauma, which produces an intrabony haematoma which fails to organise and breaks down to leave a bone cavity. However, because the same argument is used to explain why these cysts resolve after surgery, the lesion is more appropriately considered idio-pathic.

EPIDERMOID/DERMOID CYSTS

Epidermoid/dermoid cysts are soft tissue lesions which contain keratin. They are sometimes misnamed seba-ceous cysts despite the absence of a sebaceous element. Dermoid cysts contain adnexal structures such as hair follicles or sebaceous glands in their walls, whereas the more frequent epidermoid cysts do not. Both types of cyst are lined by stratified squamous epithelium which is often flattened. There is orthokera-tosis and keratin flakes fill the cyst cavity (**5.30**). Typically, no inflammation develops in the wall unless the cyst ruptures. When keratin contacts the sur-rounding tissues, it acts as an endogenous foreign body provoking a florid foreign body giant cell reaction (**5.31**).

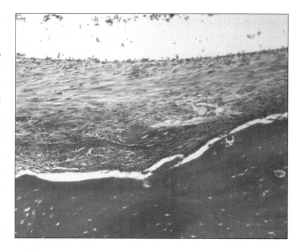

5.29 Simple bone cyst.

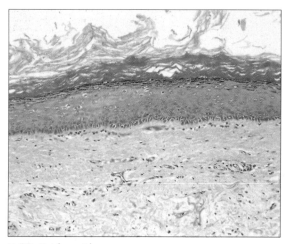

5.30 Epidermoid cyst.

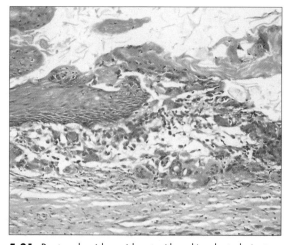

5.31 Ruptured epidermoid cyst with multinucleated giant cell foreign body reaction.

NASOPALATINE DUCT CYSTS

Nasopalatine duct (incisive canal) cysts are variable in appearance and are frequently inflamed. They may present as a swelling or be a fortuitous radiographic finding.

The wall of the nasopalatine duct cyst typically contains blood vessels and nerves (**5.32**). The cyst lining is respiratory type epithelium (particularly cysts near the nasal aspect) or stratified columnar ciliated epithelium — often with mucous cells. In other areas the lining may be squamous. Cysts near the oral cavity tend to be lined by stratified squamous epithelium. There may be combinations of both types or sometimes non-specific, flattened stratified squamous epithelium. Inflammation of the cyst wall is common.

NASOLABIAL CYSTS

Nasolabial cysts are rare soft tissue cysts which probably develop from remnants of the nasolacrimal rod or duct. They usually form a painless swelling laterally above the upper lip and may obliterate the nasolabial fold. They are lined by stratified squamous or columnar epithelium and may have foci of mucous cells (**5.33**).

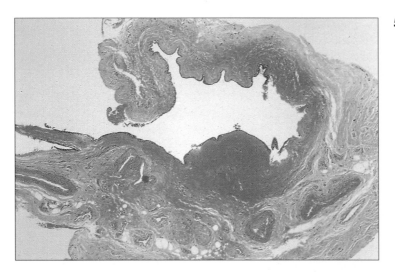

5.32 Nasopalatine duct cyst.

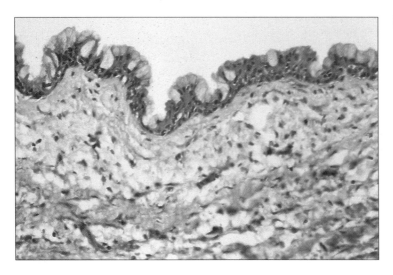

5.33 Nasolabial cyst.

6.

ODONTOGENIC TUMOURS

AMELOBLASTOMAS

The ameloblastoma is the most common odontogenic tumour. It accounts for about one per cent of all jaw tumours and is thought to originate from the cell rests of Serres. It is found mainly in the angle or ramus of the mandible. Rarely, the tumour is entirely extraosseous. Although the ameloblastoma is locally invasive and destructive it rarely metastasises. Metastatic spread is typically by aspiration although haematogenous dissemination may occasionally develop.

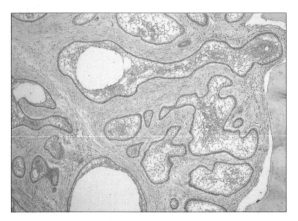

6.1 Follicular ameloblastoma.

FOLLICULAR AMELOBLASTOMAS

Follicular ameloblastomas consist of islands or follicles of odontogenic epithelium of varying sizes which infiltrate bone (**6.1**). Some follicles are distended and show central cystic degeneration. The most characteristic feature is the peripheral cells, which are palisaded, with nuclei polarised away from the typically prominent basement membrane (**6.2**). The peripheral cells are ameloblast-like but lack a Tomes' process and do not form enamel or induce changes in the adjacent connective tissue.

The central area of the follicle resembles the stellate reticulum. Its cells are often separated by intercellular oedema and microcyst formation is common. The cysts may distend and coalesce to form macrocysts which give the tumour its characteristic multilocular appearance on radiographs. The fibrous tissue stroma is bland, there is no inflammation and no tendency toward fibroblastic stroma formation.

The central area of the follicles often undergoes squamous metaplasia with the development of intercellular bridges and keratinisation. This can be florid, occasionally to the point where so much of the lesion is replaced by squamous cells that it may resemble a squamous cell carcinoma (**6.3**). Ultimately, all the islands may consist of squamous epithelium, often with flattened peripheral cells, and

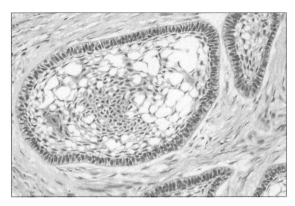

6.2 Follicular ameloblastoma (high power).

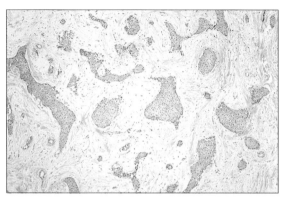

6.3 Acanthomatous ameloblastoma.

bearing little resemblance to the classical amelo-blastoma (**6.4**). This is the acanthomatous variant of ameloblastoma which can be mistaken for invasive squamous cell carcinoma. However, the squamous elements are always cytologically bland, there are no mitotic figures, or reactive changes in the connective tissue which are typical of a true squamous cell carcinoma.

PLEXIFORM AMELOBLASTOMAS

The other common variant of the ameloblastoma has a plexiform configuration. The importance of the plexiform variant is that on superficial examination it does not immediately appear to be an ameloblastoma (**6.5**). There are interconnecting strands of epithelium and cyst-forming stromal degeneration. The stellate reticulum-like areas are often minimal and the amelo-blasts are not prominent in some parts (**6.6**).

Sometimes the plexiform ameloblastoma resembles the epithelial arcades and interconnected strands seen in a periapical granuloma, except that in this case the inflammation typical of the granuloma is often absent (**6.7, 6.8**). Sometimes this is the only distinguishing feature. The plexiform type of amelo-blastoma may particularly present as a small area of mural thickening in what otherwise appears to be an odontogenic cyst.

GRANULAR CELL AMELOBLASTOMAS

The granular cell ameloblastoma is a variant which is particularly common in African people. The central cells of the follicles become rounded and granular (**6.9**). Although there is no difference in the behaviour of the tumours, they are often much larger and have a slightly different distribution to those found in the UK and the USA (where most ameloblastomas present in the angle of the mandible and expand into the ascending ramus). The granular cell ameloblastoma often presents in the anterior part of the mandible and the symphyseal region.

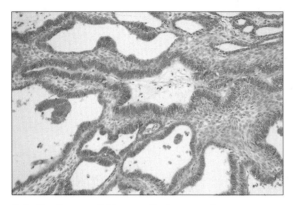

6.4 Acanthomatous ameloblastoma (higher power).

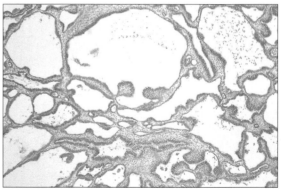

6.5 Plexiform ameloblastoma.

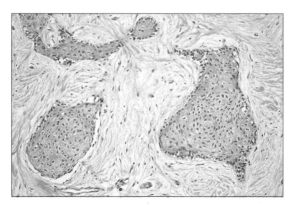

6.6 Plexiform ameloblastoma (higher power).

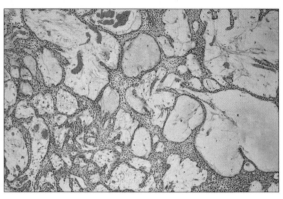

6.7 Plexiform ameloblastoma resembling epitheliated periapical granuloma.

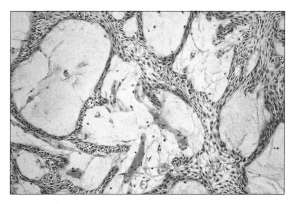

6.8 Plexiform ameloblastoma resembling epitheliated periapical granuloma (higher power).

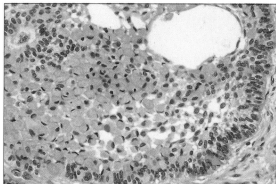

6.9 Granular cell ameloblastoma.

UNICYSTIC AMELOBLASTOMAS

Ameloblastomas can sometimes present as a unilocular cystic radiolucent area or in a pseudo-dentigerous relationship to a tooth (when the tooth has been enveloped by the tumour). Occasionally, the ameloblastoma may be in a true dentigerous relationship to the tooth (part of the cyst being attached to the amelo-cemental junction). Because the ameloblastomatous elements in some cystic tumours are minimal (and may consist of no more than a small area of mural thickening) it is important for a pathologist to scrutinise carefully any jaw cyst, pay special attention to areas of mural thickening and ensure they are sampled adequately.

In the specimen shown, part of the cyst wall, which is lined by attenuated stratified squamous epithelium, resembles a radicular cyst (**6.10**). In other areas of the specimen, the epithelium forms arcades — as might be seen in a dental cyst — but lacks inflammation. However, there are areas of budding one of which shows a distinct peripheral palisade with an ameloblastoma-like, highly prominent basement membrane and nuclei polarised away from it. An appearance such as this strongly suggests an ameloblastoma. In other parts of the specimen there were more obvious islands of ameloblastoma in the wall.

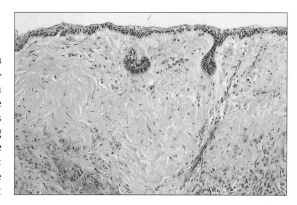

6.10 Unicystic ameloblastoma.

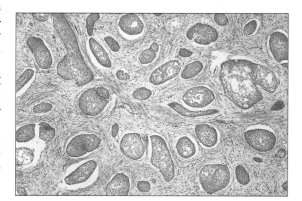

6.11 Squamous odontogenic tumour.

SQUAMOUS ODONTOGENIC TUMOURS

The squamous odontogenic tumour is uncommon and arises almost exclusively in the periodontal ligament. It consists of islands of squamous epithelium, probably odontogenic in origin, but differs from the ameloblastoma by lacking peripheral palisading and showing more of a fibroblastic response in the stroma (**6.11**). The islands of cells are all cytologically bland, in contrast to a squamous cell carcinoma. Squamous odontogenic tumours can spread into adjacent soft tissue but tend to have a benign course and not recur after removal.

ADENOMATOID ODONTOGENIC TUMOURS

The adenomatoid odontogenic tumour (formerly called adenoameloblastoma) is probably a hamartoma. This tumour arises in a younger age group and in different sites to the ameloblastoma. The majority of patients are under 20 years of age and the most common site is the maxillary canine and incisor region. It is often associated with an unerupted tooth and frequently presents as a radiolucent area, often with punctate calcifications. The adenomatoid odontogenic tumour is usually circumscribed and consists of whorls of cells which are solid or form duct-like structures (**6.12**). The cell masses are typically bilayered, consisting of a peripheral layer of palisaded cells which are ameloblast-like, and a less regular central area of cells. The two layers may be separated by eosinophilic material, frequently in the form of a thickened, convoluted band (which is thought to be a form of enamel matrix elaborated by the tumour). The duct-like structures are microcysts and arise from stromal degeneration. The basement membrane is on the luminal aspect and the cells are polarised away from the central lumen. The tumour has combinations of these two patterns. In between the formed elements are spindle-shaped cells which look like stroma but are, in fact, epithelial tumour cells. Occasionally there are focal areas of deposition of enameloid-type material or calcifications which are a form of disordered osteodentine, sometimes with tubules but usually in an irregular, haphazard arrangement.

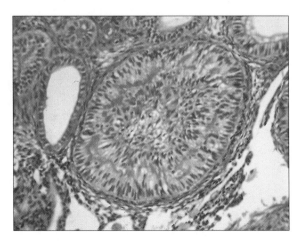

6.12 Adenomatoid odontogenic tumour.

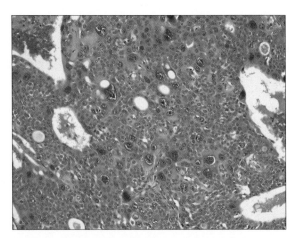

6.13 Calcifying epithelial odontogenic tumour.

CALCIFYING EPITHELIAL ODONTOGENIC TUMOURS (PINDBORG TUMOURS)

The calcifying epithelial odontogenic tumour (CEOT) is rare and typically forms a multiloculated radiolucent area with variable degrees of calcification and expansion of the bone. It can arise in either jaw but is more common in the mandible. It may be associated with an unerupted tooth.

The CEOT can have a highly variable histological appearance, which may simulate malignancy. The classical form of the tumour consists of sheets or islands of eosinophilic, polyhedral epithelial cells, often with prominent intercellular bridges, which show extensive nuclear variation (**6.13**). Giant nuclear forms and multinucleated cells may also be present (**6.14**). Although these tumours are cytologically dysplastic it is exceptionally uncommon to find mitotic figures. There can also be calcifications

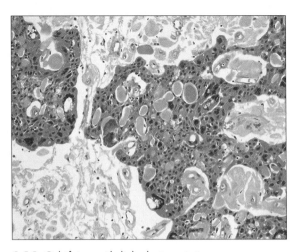

6.14 Calcifying epithelial odontogenic tumour.

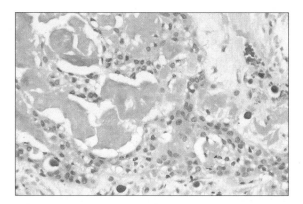

6.15 Calcifying epithelial odontogenic tumour. Congo red stain.

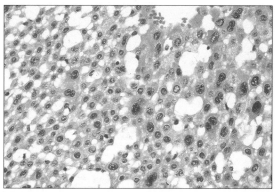

6.16 Calcifying epithelial odontogenic tumour — clear cell variant.

which are typically spheroidal and may show concentric laminations (Liesegang's rings). The material between the cells, which is pink and homogeneous, stains for amyloid with Congo red (**6.15**) and thioflavine T, a fluorescent dye.

In some CEOTs, many of the cells are clear (**6.16**). There are few multinucleated cells but some giant nuclear forms are present; there may be no calcifications. Clear cell tumours are diagnostically challenging because similar appearances can be seen in mucoepidermoid carcinomas, acinic cell carcinomas and clear cell variants of metastatic lesions from the kidney, thyroid gland and melanoma.

The CEOT is locally infiltrative with about the same growth potential as the ameloblastoma, and needs to be excised with a margin of normal bone. In common with ameloblastomas, there may be extra-osseous variants.

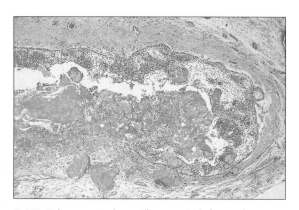

6.17 Odontogenic ghost cell tumour (calcifying odontogenic cyst).

ODONTOGENIC GHOST CELL TUMOURS (CALCIFYING ODONTOGENIC CYSTS)

These rare tumours usually produce a painless swelling and the majority arise in the mandible. Although odontogenic ghost cell tumours may be cystic, and are sometimes included in classifications of odontogenic cysts, they may be solid. The cysts and epithelial islands are lined with odontogenic epithelium with basal cell nuclei polarised away from the basement membrane, thus resembling an ameloblastoma (**6.17**). More superficially, the cells undergo an aberrant form of keratinisation and become enlarged and pale-staining (ghost cells) (**6.18**). Rupture of the cyst wall causes a florid endogenous

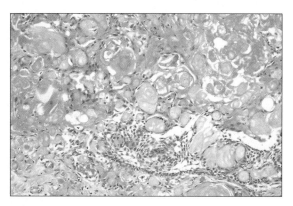

6.18 Odontogenic ghost cell tumour (calcifying odontogenic cyst) (higher power).

foreign body giant cell reaction in the surrounding tissues. Dysplastic dentine formation is common and occasionally odontomas will be associated with the tumour. Odontogenic ghost cell tumours are benign and conservative excision is curative.

AMELOBLASTIC FIBROMAS

The ameloblastic fibroma is most common at the angle of the mandible. The tumour sometimes extends for a considerable distance into the ramus even as far as the sigmoid notch. It can present at any age, but is more common in children about three to four years old. There may be associated calcification and sometimes formation of dental tissue — when the lesion becomes known as an ameloblastic fibro-odontome (**6.19**). It is controversial whether these tumours merely represent a stage in the formation of either a complex or a compound odontome. Most ameloblastic fibromas, however, do not show calcification.

The ameloblastomic fibroma epithelium resembles that of an ameloblastoma but the follicles usually have a more uniform structure and most of the islands show striking reversed polarity (**6.20, 6.21**). Microcyst formation may develop in the stellate reticulum-like area but this is less common and less extensive than in follicular ameloblastomas and there is no squamous metaplasia. There may be granular cell change, but this is typically in the stroma rather than in the follicles.

The stroma is a mesenchymal tissue which resembles primitive dental pulp and is therefore distinct from the stroma of other odontogenic tumours. It is very cellular and shows little collagen formation. In contrast, the stromal component of an odontogenic fibroma is virtually fibrous. Although the ameloblastic fibroma is a benign tumour it can recur. It is important to exclude the malignant variant, the ameloblastic sarcoma, by examining the stroma carefully for any nuclear pleomorphism or mitotic activity. Although the ameloblastic sarcoma is of low grade malignancy, it is locally destructive and occasionally metastasises. However, young people with a growing ameloblastic fibroma inevitably show some degree of mitotic activity which often renders interpretation difficult.

ODONTOGENIC FIBROMAS

The odontogenic fibroma is not a single lesion but represents a poorly characterised group of odontogenic tumours. Some pathologists believe that hyperplastic tooth follicles are examples of odontogenic fibromas but it is debatable at which point a hyperplastic lesion becomes a frank tumour.

There are two main types of odontogenic fibroma. One resembles the dental follicle and usually has rather sparse epithelial elements (**6.22**). The other type has more epithelial elements and occasionally substantial calcification and other changes (**6.23, 6.24**).

6.19 Ameloblastic fibro-odontome.

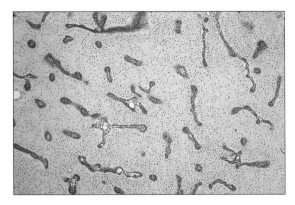

6.20 Ameloblastic fibroma.

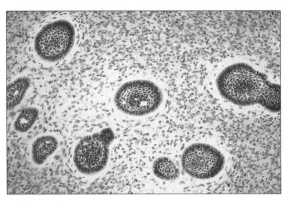

6.21 Ameloblastic fibroma.

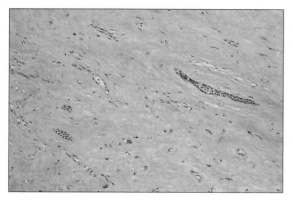

6.22 Odontogenic fibroma.

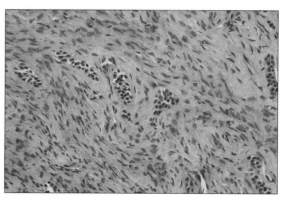

6.23 Odontogenic fibroma.

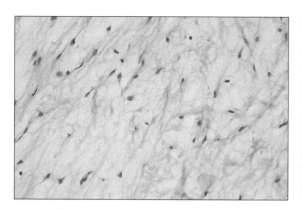

6.24 Odontogenic fibroma with calcifications.

ODONTOGENIC MYXOMAS

These are rare tumours which are exclusive to the jaws and typically present in young people. They form a slow growing swelling and related teeth may loosen or drift. Odontogenic myxomas are frequently associated with a missing tooth and characteristic soap-bubble like areas of radiolucency. Microscopy shows mucoid, basophilic ground substance with scanty angular or stellate cells (**6.25, 6.26**). There is variable collagenisation — tumours with plentiful fibrous tissue are termed fibromyxomas. Occasionally there may be strands or foci of odontogenic epithelium. The tumour is benign but has a tendency to recur due to incomplete removal (because the limits of the tumour are often difficult to define).

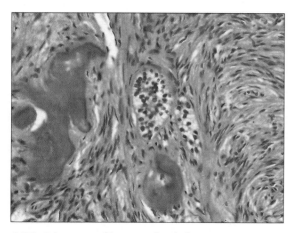

6.25 Odontogenic myxoma.

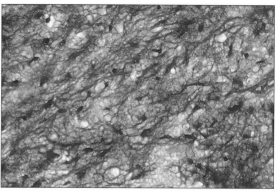

6.26 Odontogenic myxoma. Alcian blue stain.

COMPLEX ODONTOMES

Complex odontomes are usually single lesions replacing, or seen in addition to, normal teeth. They usually present as a densely radio-opaque mass and consist of a haphazard mixture of dental tissues, predominantly dentine. At low power, the most obvious feature is calcified tissue, most of which is dentine with multiple spaces where the enamel has dissolved out during decalcification (leaving fragments of enamel matrix) (**6.27**). At high power, the prismatic structure of the immature enamel matrix can be seen.

In addition to the irregular mass of dental tissue there may be areas of odontogenic epithelium which are the remnants of the formative tissue. Some odontomes erupt into the mouth which results in secondary inflammatory changes.

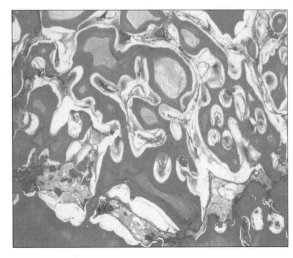

6.27 Complex odontome.

COMPOUND ODONTOMES

Compound odontomes consist of an encapsulated mass of discrete tooth-like denticles in a fibrous connective tissue stroma (**6.28**). In decalcified sections, the shrunken enamel organic matrix can be seen in spaces while the dentine and pulpal tissue have a relatively normal relationship. It is not uncommon for odontomes to show a combination of compound and complex types.

BENIGN CEMENTOBLASTOMAS (TRUE CEMENTOMAS)

The benign cementoblastoma is probably the only true tumour of cementum. It is an important odontogenic tumour because it can be readily mistaken for other lesions, particularly in fragmented specimens. It usually arises on the root of a lower molar or premolar tooth and forms a radio-opaque mass resorbing and attached to the root. Typically there is a radiolucent border around the radio-opaque mass which helps to differentiate it from many other lesions.

The lesion consists of an irregular mass of calcified tissue, which is dense with very little interstitial material. One of the most striking features is a basophilic resting and reversal line pattern which resembles the so-called mosaic pattern of Paget's disease (**6.29**). The other main feature of the benign cementoblastoma is cells which are often large and pleomorphic, and can appear cytologically malignant. Some of these cells resemble plump osteoblasts while

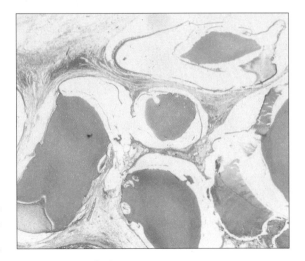

6.28 Compound odontome.

others are multinucleated (**6.30**). The appearance of these large cells and multinucleated cells resorbing the cementum might reinforce the misconception that the lesion is Paget's disease or, in some cases, because they are so bizarre, the possibility of osteo-sarcoma.

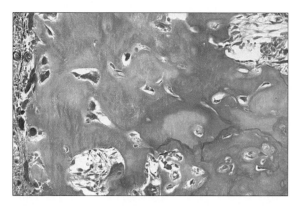

6.29 Benign cementoblastoma.

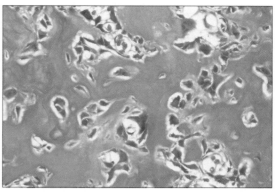

6.30 Benign cementoblastoma.

CEMENTIFYING FIBROMA (CEMENTO-OSSIFYING FIBROMA) AND PERIAPICAL CEMENTAL DYSPLASIA

Cementifying fibroma and periapical cemental dysplasia are probably the same condition, but they are said to have one or two clinically distinguishing features. Typically, periapical cemental dysplasia affects several teeth, most commonly in the lower incisor region, whereas cementifying fibromas tend to affect a single tooth, usually in the molar region. Periapical cemental dysplasia tends to be seen in young people while cementifying fibroma affects older individuals.

The normal sequence of events in the development of periapical cemental dysplasia is the appearance of a radiolucent area around the root of one or several teeth which resembles a periapical granuloma (the teeth, however, remain vital). There is progressive calcification which, radiographically, is initially punctate. Eventually the whole mass becomes radio-opaque, but not in continuity with the root of the tooth. The same happens in cementifying fibroma — a periapical radiolucency (which is usually greater than occurs in periapical cemental dysplasia) shows progressive calcification ultimately forming a radio-opaque mass, again not attached to the root of the tooth. The tooth retains vitality. The two lesions are often indistinguishable histologically, and the features are the same as those seen in both ossifying fibroma and fibrous dysplasia (**6.31**).

In some cases the calcified tissue is laid down in laminated, spheroidal masses which resemble cemticles (**6.32**) although it is uncommon for large areas of the lesion to show this appearance.

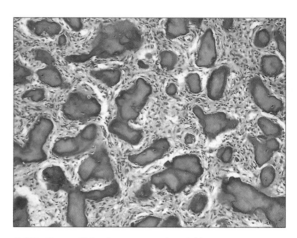

6.31 Cementifying (cemento-ossifying) fibroma.

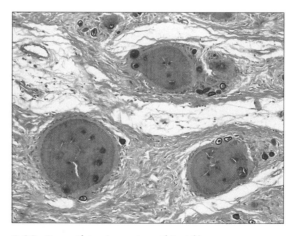

6.32 Cementifying (cemento-ossifying) fibroma.

FLORID CEMENTO-OSSEOUS DYSPLASIA (GIGANTIFORM CEMENTOMA)

Florid cemento-osseous dysplastic lesions are usually multiple and may involve all four quadrants, typically in middle-aged black females. They produce slow growing painless swellings but there may be ulceration of the overlying mucosa and secondary osteomyelitis. Radiographs show diffuse, dense areas of radiopacity. Microscopy shows acellular masses of dense calcified tissue (osteo-cementum) (**6.33**). These lesions are considered to be dysplastic rather than neoplastic.

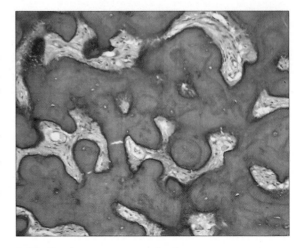

6.33 Florid cemento-osseous dysplasia.

7.

BONE

ACUTE OSTEOMYELITIS OF THE JAW

The bone is necrotic in acute osteomyelitis. Dead bone is recognised histologically as it does not contain osteocytes in the osteocyte lacunae. The affected bone shows irregular areas of resorption and is surrounded by vascular, haemorrhagic, acute and chronically inflamed tissue — sometimes containing islands of bacteria (**7.1**). The interstitial tissue consists predominantly of granulation tissue, attempting repair. In addition, there may be foci of osteoclastic resorption. In osteomyelitis of the jaws, however, there is often limited involucrum formation.

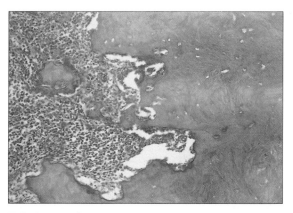

7.1 Osteomyelitis.

PULSE GRANULOMAS (HYALINE RING GRANULOMAS; GIANT CELL PERIOSTITIS)

This uncommon condition usually produces a tender swelling in the posterior part of the edentulous alveolar mucosa. There may be evidence of erosion of the underlying bone. Microscopy shows eosinophilic rings of hyaline material surrounded by chronic inflammatory cells and multinucleated giant cells (**7.2**). The rings can be incomplete and may surround giant cells or vessels. The rings are thought to be vegetable in nature and are probably cooked pulses with collagen deposits on their surface.

FIBROUS DYSPLASIA

Fibrous dysplasia is a fibro-osseous lesion that can affect one (monostotic) or several (polystotic) bones. Progressive swelling develops which typically stabilises around puberty. The maxilla is the most commonly affected site in the head and neck region.

The classical microscopic features of fibrous dysplasia are bone resorption followed by replacement with moderately cellular fibrous tissue within which metaplastic, coarse woven bone is deposited in thin, slender spicules forming a characteristic 'Chinese letter pattern' arrangement (**7.3**). The bone does not show osteones and rarely any osteoid. The fibrous

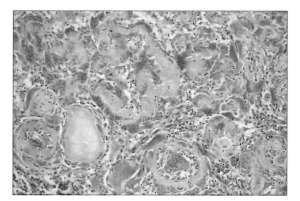

7.2 Pulse granuloma.

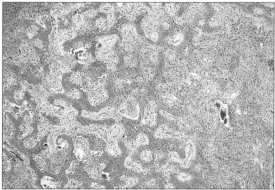

7.3 Fibrous dysplasia.

connective tissue is typically non-inflamed and rarely vascular (**7.4**). Virtually identical appearances are seen in some areas of cementifying fibroma and in periapical cemental dysplasia. Sometimes there are focal areas of multinucleated giant cells in fibrous dysplasia, typically in relation to areas of haemorrhage and occasionally in relation to resorbing bone.

OSSIFYING FIBROMAS

Ossifying fibromas can be distinguished from fibrous dysplasia clinically and radiologically although their histological features are similar. Whereas fibrous dysplasia typically arrests at skeletal maturation, ossifying fibromas may continue to grow after that age or commence growth in adult life. Radiographically, fibrous dysplasia shows an area of diffuse radiolucency classically giving a ground glass or orange peel appearance. Ossifying fibromas form a discrete radiolucent area often with a sclerotic margin and contain variable radio-opaque masses. Ossifying fibromas can be locally aggressive in long bones although in the jaws they tend to progress slowly and gradually calcify.

Histologically it may not be possible to differentiate the ossifying fibroma from any of the fibro-osseous lesions just described. The histological appearance illustrated is typical and shows an outer shell of lamellar bone laid down in sheets and deeper woven bone (**7.5**). Cellular fibrous tissue with calcified spherules exist in the deepest part of the lesion (**7.6**).

It must be emphasised that fibro-osseous lesions are **clinico-pathological diagnoses** rather than purely histological diagnoses.

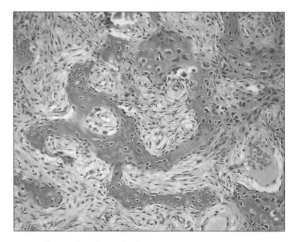

7.4 Fibrous dysplasia (higher power).

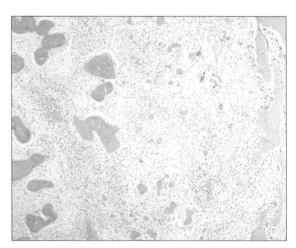

7.5 Ossifying fibroma.

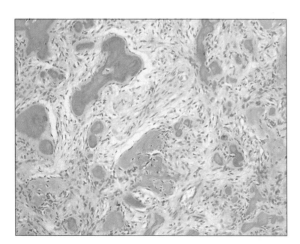

7.6 Ossifying fibroma.

CHERUBISM

Although cherubism has been called familial fibrous dysplasia, it has few similarities histologically or clinically to typical fibrous dysplasia. Cherubism usually presents as swellings of the mandible, particularly at the angle and the ramus although sometimes there are swellings in the maxilla. The jaw swellings produce very characteristic bilateral multiloculated radiolucent areas and biopsy shows variable amounts of fibrous tissue and giant cells. It predominantly presents in males between the ages of about two to four years.

Microscopy shows multinucleated giant cells in a vascular fibroblastic stroma, an appearance which cannot be distinguished from central giant cell granulomas or hyperparathyroidism on histology alone

(**7.7**). Cherubism is a clinico-pathological diagnosis, **not** a histological one. One supposedly typical histological feature is collagen deposition around vessels to produce an eosinophilic or hyaline cuff. However, it is impossible to rely on this feature to make the diagnosis as it is relatively uncommon. Significant new bone formation is rare — a feature which does help to differentiate cherubism from fibrous dysplasia.

There may also be cervical lymphadenopathy, which is reactive (presumably from draining an area where there is interstitial haemorrhage). Typically, cherubism arrests around about the age of puberty, or slightly later, and often resolves with considerable remodelling of the jaws. However, radiographs can often provide evidence of quiescent disease — even years afterwards.

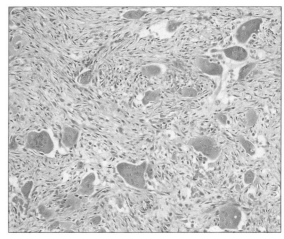

7.7 Cherubism.

CENTRAL GIANT CELL GRANULOMAS

These destructive lesions of bone affect the mandible more commonly than the maxilla and are typically seen in patients between the ages of 10–25 years. They may be symptomless or cause a swelling of the bone. Occasionally there may be pain, mental nerve or infraorbital paraesthesia or anaesthesia, and loosening of teeth. Radiographs show an ill-defined area of radiolucency sometimes with root displacement or resorption. Microscopy shows multinucleated, osteoclast-like giant cells in a vascular stroma of plump, spindle-shaped cells which may show mitotic figures (**7.8, 7.9**). The giant cells may be evenly scattered or aggregated around foci of haemorrhage. Occasionally giant cells appear to be within vascular spaces. There is frequent osseous metaplasia and/or dystrophic calcification within the stroma.

These features are not diagnostic and similar histological changes can be seen in areas of aneurysmal bone cysts, cherubism and hyperparathyroidism.

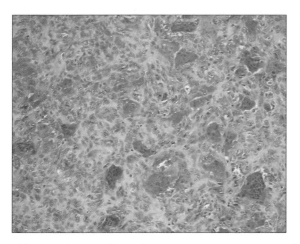

7.8 Central giant cell granuloma.

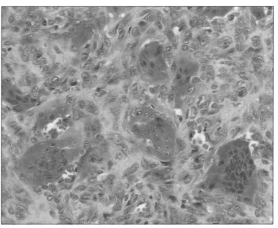

7.9 Central giant cell granuloma (higher power).

HYPERPARATHYROIDISM

The brown tumours of hyperparathyroidism are giant cell lesions which are impossible to differentiate histologically from many of the other giant cell lesions which affect the jaw. The specimens show multinucleated giant cells in a fibroblastic, vascular stroma, with areas of haemorrhage and haemosiderin deposition (**7.10**). The diagnosis can only be confirmed by biochemical means, i.e. demonstrating elevated blood calcium, normal or low phosphate and raised alkaline phosphatase levels.

PAGET'S DISEASE OF BONE

Paget's disease is characterised by an uncoordinated apposition and resorption of bone without regard to normal functional requirements. Its frequency increases over the age of 40 years and lesions typically involve the pelvis, long bones and calvarium of the skull. Jaw involvement is uncommon but is seen most frequently in the maxilla as a slow growing enlargement and deformity.

The specimen shown (**7.11**) illustrates bone being laid down and resorbed in a completely irregular and haphazard manner, within a very vascular stroma. Patchy inflammation is sometimes seen in the stroma, and the bone may reveal basophilic reversal lines where there has been a repetitive sequence of resorption and deposition (**7.12**). This produces a so-called mosaic pattern which is really more like a jigsaw in that the pieces are not square (as in a mosaic) but typically 'Mickey Mouse ear' shaped.

The bone is initially vital but in later stages there is dense sclerosis and vitality becomes compromised.

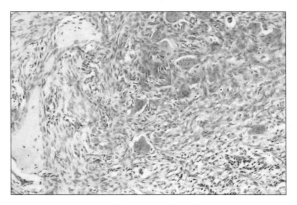

7.10 Brown tumour of hyperparathyroidism.

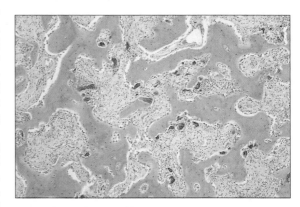

7.11 Paget's disease of bone.

OSTEOMAS

Osteomas can either be compact or cancellous. They are usually subperiosteal although endosteal osteomas can form. The latter are rare and most reported cases have been misdiagnoses — being other lesions such as dense bone islands, cementomas, areas of focal chronic sclerosing osteomyelitis, or sometimes simply a piece of tooth root. The example shown is a true endosteal osteoma (thus growing within the bone) and consists of dense mature bone with Haversian systems (osteones) (**7.13**).

Cancellous osteomas consist of trabeculae of lamellar bone and variable amounts of fibrofatty marrow tissue (**7.14**).

Multiple osteomas of the jaws are a feature of Gardner's syndrome (an autosomal dominant inherited trait) when they are associated with multiple fibrous tumours and sebaceous cysts of the skin. Colonic polyposis, which may undergo malignant change in early adult life, is also a feature of this syndrome.

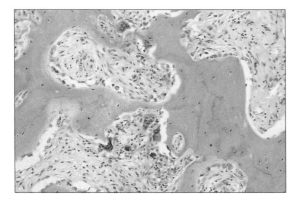

7.12 Paget's disease of bone.

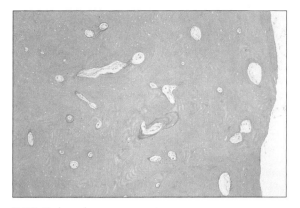

7.13 Endosteal osteoma.

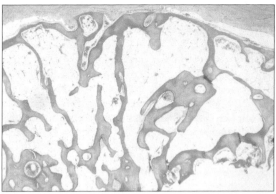

7.14 Cancellous osteoma.

OSTEOSARCOMA

The essential feature of an osteosarcoma is the formation of malignant bone by a sarcomatous stroma. Osteosarcomas rarely form the classical sunray appearance on radiographs (typical of tumours of long bones) in the jaws.

In this example, irregular osteoid is shown with pleomorphic cells in the stroma. The malignant osteoblasts (which would stain for alkaline phosphatase) are irregularly disposed (**7.15**). There are excess numbers of mitoses and other cytological features of malignancy such as pleomorphism and a high nuclear–cytoplasmic ratio. In addition, there are giant forms and multinucleated tumour cells (**7.16**). In osteosarcomas of the jaw, extensive cartilage formation is common (so-called chondroblastic osteosarcoma) (**7.17**).

Some osteosarcomas contain many multinucleated giant cells and it is probably this variant which is sometimes confused with the so-called true giant cell tumours of the jaws.

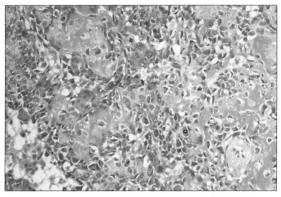

7.15 Osteosarcoma.

Osteosarcomas widely metastasise via the blood to the lung at an early stage, which results in the typically poor prognosis. In the head and neck region, however, local extension of tumour is often the more clinically significant problem.

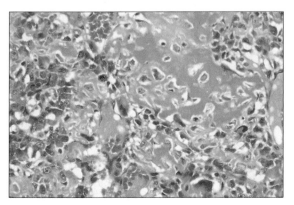

7.16 Osteosarcoma (higher power).

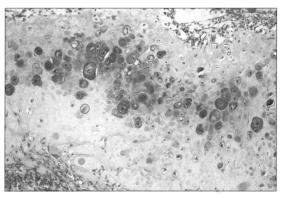

7.17 Chondroblastic osteosarcoma.

CHONDROMAS AND CHONDRO-SARCOMAS

Chondroblastic tumours tend to arise in those parts of the jaw where there is normally cartilage, such as the condyle, coronoid process, and symphyseal region of the mandible, and the anterior part of the maxilla. The distinction between benign and malignant cartilaginous tumours is histologically difficult and may, at times, prove impossible.

Typically the tumour is lobulated, and usually cellular (**7.18, 7.19**). One of the main features that differentiates chondrosarcoma from chondroma is the presence of multiple nuclei in some of the sarcoma cells. Bizarre nuclei, however, are common in most cartilaginous tumours because cartilaginous cells tend to swell and degenerate. The nuclear configura-tion, mitoses, evidence of invasion and absence of osteoid formation characterise chondrosarcomas (**7.20**). If there is osteoid formation in the tumour it is likely to be a chondroblastic osteosarcoma. The main difficulty with the diagnosis of chondrosarcomas is to differentiate them from osteosarcoma and chondroma. As the cytological features of benign cartilaginous tumours can be rather bizarre, many pathologists tend to rely on site rather than the histology when making the distinction. For example, a great deal of pleomorphism may be accepted in a cartilaginous tumour of the finger, because most cartilaginous tumours of the finger are benign. However, the same degree of atypia in a cartilaginous tumour of the vertebra would cause alarm because most cartilaginous tumours of the vertebra are malignant. In the jaws, it can thus be very difficult to make a distinction.

Chondrosarcomas are usually slow-growing and produce local recurrences (it is very easy to seed the wound with tumour during attempted excision). Metastasis tends to be a late event, usually after several recurrences. However, jaw chondrosarcomas have a very poor prognosis due to the involvement of local vital structures.

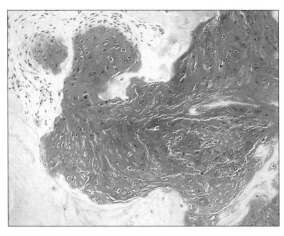

7.18 Chondrosarcoma invading bone.

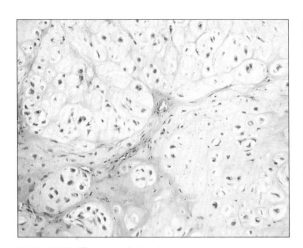

7.19 Well-differentiated chondrosarcoma.

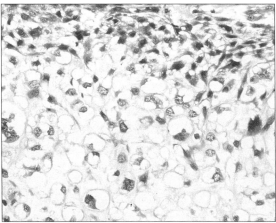

7.20 Pleomorphism in chondrosarcoma.

EOSINOPHILIC GRANULOMAS (LANGERHANS' CELL HISTIO-CYTOSES)

This is a rare disease characterised by solitary or multiple osteolytic lesions. It is part of a spectrum of lesions formally known as histiocytosis X — now termed Langerhans' cell histiocytosis. The main types are solitary eosinophilic granuloma, multifocal eosinophilic granuloma (including Hand-Schuller-Christian disease) and Letter Siwe disease (progressive disseminated histiocytosis). There is proliferation of Langerhans' cells which can be identified with electron microscopy by characteristic rod- or racquet-shaped Birbeck granules or immunocytochemical staining for S100 protein or peanut agglutinin lectin.

Microscopy of eosinophilic granuloma (solitary or multifocal) shows pale histiocytes with lobulated or indented nuclei which produces a coffee-bean-like appearance (**7.21**, **7.22**). In addition, there are variable numbers of eosinophils. In resolving or treated lesions there may be progressive fibrosis.

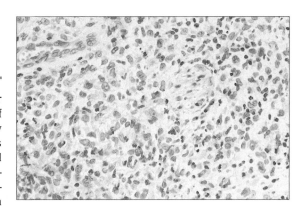

7.21 Eosinophilic granuloma.

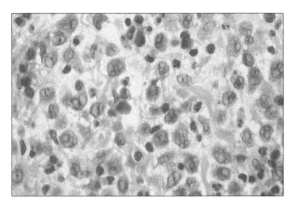

7.22 Eosinophilic granuloma (higher power).

ACTINOMYCOSIS

Cervicofacial actinomycosis is caused by the filamentous bacterium *Actinomycosis israelii* and other actinomyces and related species. Nowadays most cases present as a single indurated swelling over the mandible or upper neck, often with one or several skin sinuses. Involvement of bone is very uncommon but occasionally colonies of actinomyces are seen in specimens taken from periapical granulomas and tonsillar crypts, but these are probably of no clinical significance.

The typical lesions of actinomycosis are characterised microscopically by acute inflammation and areas of fibrous repair. Colonies of organisms form a mycelium (sulphur granule) surrounded by polymorphs, foamy macrophages and occasionally multinucleated giant cells (**7.23**, **7.24**). The mycelium is Gram-positive and sometimes Gram-negative clubs of lipid can be seen in the host tissue at the periphery of the colony.

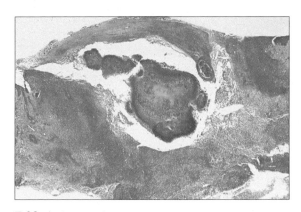

7.23 Actinomycosis.

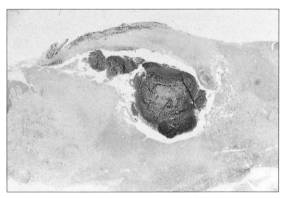

7.24 Actinomycosis. Gram stain.

8.
GRANULOMATOUS LESIONS

SARCOIDOSIS

Sarcoidosis is an idiopathic chronic disease characterised by the formation of non-caseating epithelioid granulomas in multiple sites including the lungs, liver, lymph nodes, skin, eyes and bones.

The granulomas in sarcoidosis are typically separated and discrete (**8.1**) whereas the granulomas in tuberculosis tend to fuse and form conglomerate follicles. The multinucleated giant cells related to the epithelioid granulomas in sarcoidosis are usually scattered; the amount of inflammation is variable. Sarcoid granulomas tend to heal by fibrosis.

In some cases of sarcoidosis the giant cells contain crystalline inclusions which are usually concentrically laminated (Schaumann bodies) (**8.2**) or star-shaped (asteroid bodies). These inclusions, although most commonly seen in sarcoidosis, are not diagnostic.

The serum level of angiotensin converting enzyme, which is produced predominantly by pulmonary macrophages, may be raised in sarcoidosis and there is usually some degree of either interstitial pulmonary involvement or bilateral hilar lymphadenopathy visible on a chest radiograph. A granulomatous condition affecting the mouth associated with bilateral hilar lymphadenopathy almost guarantees this diagnosis. The other test which was frequently used in the past was the Kveim test. This involved injecting a sterilised tissue extract, usually prepared from the spleen of a patient with sarcoidosis, into the dermis (typically the forearm) and excising the area six to twelve weeks later to seek evidence of sarcoid granulomas. This specimen shows the skin overlying a florid granulomatous reaction and represents a typical positive Kveim reaction (**8.3**). The main problem with the Kveim reaction is that the reagent itself is variable in reactivity (because it comes from patients) and there is an additional need for caution with the technique. For example, the use of plastic syringes results in a foreign body giant cell reaction (due to the presence of the silicone grease lubricant) which necessitates the use of glass syringes. Furthermore, if the needle is inserted too deeply and enters the underlying subcutaneous fat, necrosis may result — a giant cell granulomatous reaction. The specificity of the test is also not

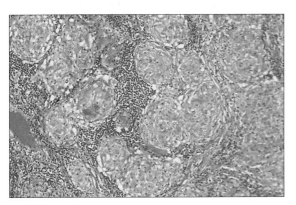

8.1 Sarcoidosis.

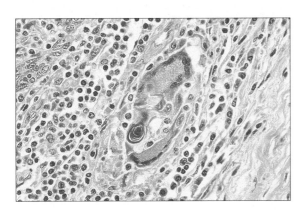

8.2 Sarcoidosis — Schaumann body in multinucleated giant cell.

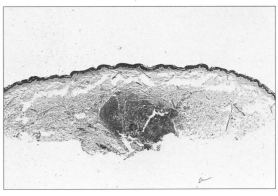

8.3 Sarcoidosis — Kveim reaction.

entire because positive Kveim reactions may be seen in conditions such as Crohn's disease. Finally, as the test requires the use of a biopsy, it is not generally performed on a routine basis.

TUBERCULOSIS

Oral tuberculosis typically presents as a single ulcer, often in the midline of the dorsum of the tongue or palate. Tuberculous ulcers are painful and have undermined, irregular margins and watery granulations in the floor (**8.4**). This example shows the undermined edge of a tuberculous ulcer. This appearance, however, can also be seen in any other ulcerative granulomatous conditions, for example, orofacial granulomatosis. The surface of the tuberculous ulcer is covered with slough (fibrin and polymorphs) while in the deeper tissue aggregates of pale staining

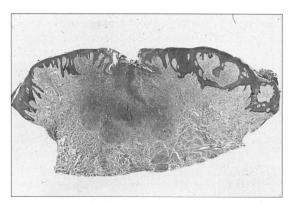

8.4 Tuberculous ulcer.

epithelioid cells — which resemble epithelial cells — can be seen (**8.5**). These are macrophages which, having lost their ability to migrate, become aggregated in sheets. They also become much more eosinophilic than normal. Because they are pink-stained and aggregated together, the macrophages resemble epithelium. Multinucleated giant cells, so-called Langhans' type giant cells, which have nuclei polarised at either end of the cell are also typically seen. However, Langhans' giant cells are certainly not specific for tuberculosis (or for any other disease).

The granulomas often fuse to form so-called conglomerate follicles. The tubercle granulomas do not usually caseate in the oral mucosa or skin.

The tuberculous granuloma is usually an effective defence mechanism: macrophages readily ingest the tubercle bacillus but the waxy coat inhibits digestion of the organisms. Cell-mediated defences include lymphocytes that produce cytokines such as macrophage migration inhibition factor and fibroblast activating factors (which eventually sequesters the bacilli in a fibrous sac). In the absence of this defence mechanism the macrophages would tend to migrate and die, releasing (and spreading) the bacilli. However, this fibrosis is responsible for much of the clinical damage as the tubercle bacillus itself is almost non-toxic.

Staining for acid–alcohol fast bacilli with a Ziehl Neelsen stain is rarely helpful in cutaneous and mucosal tuberculosis because the bacilli are very sparse. Fluorescent dyes, auramine and rhodamine, can be used to stain the tubercle bacilli which can then be visualised by a fluorescent microscope.

The main implication of finding a tuberculous ulcer is that they are virtually always accompanied by open pulmonary tuberculosis rendering the

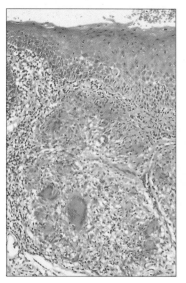

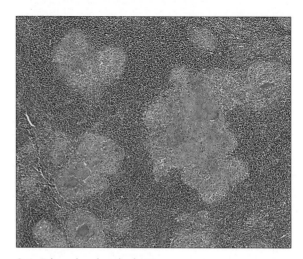

8.5 Tuberculosis (higher power).

8.6 Tuberculous lymphadenitis.

patient potentially infectious (and possibly having rapidly progressing disease).

Although bacilli should be sought, failure to isolate them does not negate the diagnosis of tuberculosis. In all suspected cases a chest radiograph must be taken.

Tuberculous cervical lymphadenitis is seen as part of a primary complex in head and neck tuberculosis. The Ghon focus is found in the tonsil and the organisms spread to the regional lymph node, which in this case is the jugulo-digastric (tonsillar) node. Discrete and coalescing epithelioid granulomas exist within the substance of the lymph node with central areas of caseation (**8.6**).

OROFACIAL GRANULOMATOSIS/ ORAL CROHN'S DISEASE

The histological appearances of orofacial granulomatosis and oral Crohn's disease are identical although the degree of inflammatory infiltration and granuloma formation is extremely variable. The most obvious feature is the presence of pronounced oedema in the papillary corium — in some areas there is fibrin exudation and dilatation of the superficial lymphatics (**8.7**). In other areas there is a patchy chronic inflammatory cell infiltration (which is predominantly lymphocytic and, to a lesser extent, plasmacytic). Most of these changes are in the superficial part of the lesion but may extend deeply into the muscle. The granulomas are usually poorly formed and have an indiscrete edge which lacks a well-defined lymphocytic cuff or fibrosis. Multinucleated giant cells are also frequently scattered or absent (**8.8**). The granulomas can either bulge into or occasionally lie free in the lymphatics. They may block the lymph drainage (endovasal granulomatous lymphangiitis) (**8.9**) producing oedema — a feature which is common in oral Crohn's disease but much less frequent in other sites, particularly rectal Crohn's disease.

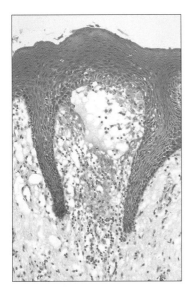

8.7 Orofacial granulomatosis.

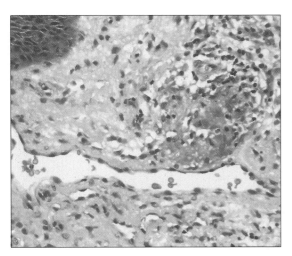

8.8 Orofacial granulomatosis.

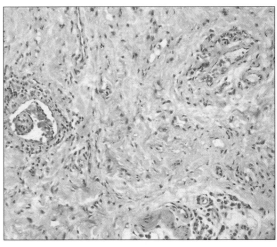

8.9 Endovasal granulomatous lymphangiitis.

FOREIGN BODY REACTION

Foreign body giant cell reactions may arise in a variety of situations in the orofacial tissues. They can be due to exogenous foreign bodies or endogenous foreign bodies — such as keratin (in relation to tumours or cysts) or bone. Endogenous foreign bodies also arise from the presence of cholesterol crystals which are irritant and produce a florid foreign body giant cell reaction.

This slide shows a granulomatous reaction to minute fragments of glass from a windscreen following a road traffic accident (**8.10**). There is a florid granulomatous reaction out of all proportion to the amount of foreign material. This type of foreign body material would show strong birefringence in polarised light. It may be important to exclude the possibility that the patient has sarcoidosis with an exaggerated foreign body reaction of this type.

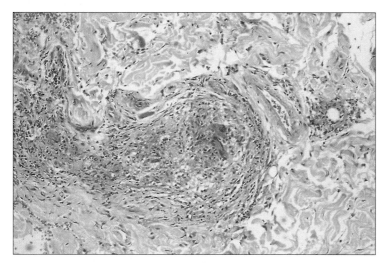

8.10 Foreign body giant cell reaction.

9.

STOMATITIS

MEDIAN RHOMBOID GLOSSITIS

Median rhomboid glossitis is typically seen as a lozenge-shaped, flat or sometimes bosselated, swelling in the midline of the tongue anterior to the sulcus terminalis. It is either red or speckled and is said to be due to persistence of one of the midline eminences present in the tongue during embryological development — the tuberculum impar. However, it is very rarely seen in children, which would not support such a hypothesis, and presents with increasing frequency with age. Smoking predisposes to this disorder and it appears to be associated

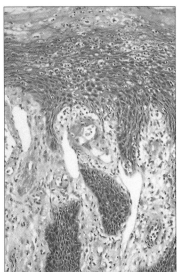

9.1 Median rhomboid glossitis.

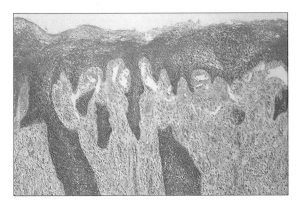

9.2 Median rhomboid glossitis (higher power).

with candidal infection. Median rhomboid glossitis can also be seen in HIV infection which also predisposes to candidosis.

The main importance of median rhomboid glossitis, apart from its occasional HIV association, is that it may (clinically and histologically) simulate malignancy.

In the example shown, the epithelium is both hyperplastic and hyperparakeratotic. There are downgrowths of rete ridges into the underlying connective tissue which are fusing (**9.1**). In addition, there are polymorphs in the superficial parakeratinised epithelium, a feature which always suggests the presence of *Candida* (**9.2**). There may be a band of hyalinised and structureless connective tissue between the corium and the underlying muscle. This is a common feature which stains for collagen and not amyloid, for which it is sometimes mistaken.

HERPES SIMPLEX

It is uncommon to biopsy either primary or recurrent herpes simplex lesions. In the early stages, there is intercellular oedema (spongiosis) with ballooning degeneration of the epithelial cells due to intracellular oedema. This eventually leads to intraepithelial vesiculation as shown (**9.3**). In common with other viral infections of the oral mucosa, multinucleated

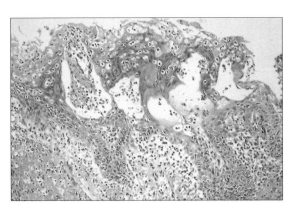

9.3 Herpes simplex vesiculation.

epithelial cells are often found (**9.4**). Eosinophilic intranuclear inclusion bodies (Lipschutz bodies) are rarely seen.

The vesicles rupture to leave shallow ulcers, typically with sharply defined margins and covered with fibrinous slough.

PEMPHIGUS VULGARIS

Pemphigus is an autoimmune disorder affecting stratified squamous epithelium, in which antibodies are directed against intercellular adhesion molecules.

Pemphigus vulgaris results in suprabasal acantholysis, in which the cells of the epithelium separate. Typically the affected cells become smaller and rounder and may be seen directly attached to the wall of the blister or floating free within it (**9.5**). There is a layer of basal cells still attached to the underlying connective tissue (tombstone cells) and a suprabasal split (**9.6**). This slide shows an obviously fresh split because there is very little associated inflammation. Occasionally, the acantholysis may be more extensive and associated with florid acute inflammatory changes (**9.7**). The Nikolsky phenomenon (from knife friction drawing across the tissue during biopsy) is often sufficient to cause the epithelium to lift off completely and be separated or lost. However, it is usually still possible to make a putative diagnosis of pemphigus by the layer of basal cells remaining attached to the connective tissue. This is because the autoantibody is directed against desmosomes while the cells remain attached to the connective tissue by hemi-desmosomes. A hemi-desmosome is not simply half a desmosome but has different antigenic properties and is not damaged by the pemphigus autoantibody. Direct or indirect immunofluorescence in frozen tissue shows intercellular antibodies and is used to confirm the diagnosis (**9.8**).

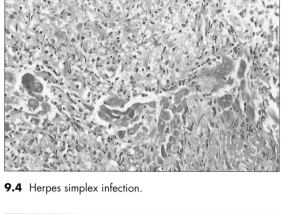

9.4 Herpes simplex infection.

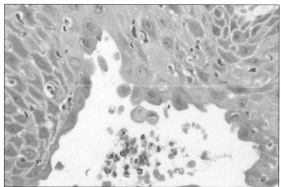

9.5 Pemphigus vulgaris showing acantholytic cells.

The cells in pemphigus vulgaris eventually separate from each other completely, distinguishing the condition from Hailey–Hailey disease (benign chronic familial pemphigus) during which some degree of intercellular cohesion is retained.

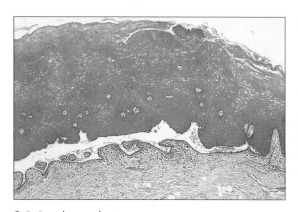

9.6 Pemphigus vulgaris.

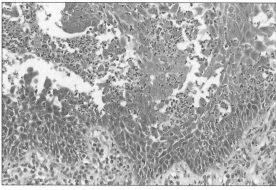

9.7 Pemphigus vulgaris.

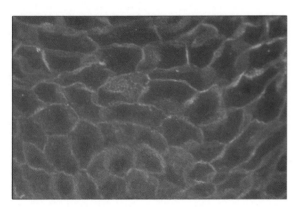

9.8 Pemphigus vulgaris — immunofluorescent staining IgG in intercellular areas.

LICHEN PLANUS

Lichen planus is a fairly common idiopathic condition affecting stratified squamous epithelia and is essentially a low power microscopical diagnosis. Many textbooks suggest that the epithelium shows irregular acanthosis, which is said to be saw-toothed, but in practice this is uncommon in oral biopsies which tend to show atrophy and hyperkeratosis. The latter can either be parakeratosis or, occasionally, orthokeratosis. Skin lichen planus more typically shows orthokeratosis or hyperkeratosis with a prominent granular cell layer, which is often focally thickened. However, this is unusual in oral lichen planus. Similarly, a saw-toothed rete ridge pattern is much more typical of skin involvement than oral disease.

A prominent rete ridge pattern is shown here, but it is not particularly saw-toothed (**9.9**). The epithelium is parakeratinised. At this power a very dense and band-like infiltrate of inflammatory cells, which are staining intensely blue, can be seen beneath the epithelium. The infiltrate predominantly consists of lymphocytes and histiocytes. There are focal areas where the junction between the inflammatory infiltrate and the epithelium is indistinct, and there are clear spaces following basal cell liquefaction (**9.10**). Civatte, or colloid bodies, which are degenerating epithelial cells, appear as eosinophilic structureless masses usually in the lower part of the epithelium or the upper part of the corium. Civatte bodies are coated with immunoglobulin and stain intensely with fluorescent anti-immunoglobulin (Ig) antibody. It is also common to have pigment loss from the damaged basal cells. The released melanin pigment is then ingested by macrophages (melanophages) (**9.11**).

This pigmentary incontinence is seen in other conditions characterised by basal cell liquefaction, such as discoid lupus erythematosus, and may also be a feature of smoker's keratosis.

There may occasionally be a conspicuous thickening of the basement membrane zone which, although usually regarded as a feature of discoid lupus erythematosus, may be seen in lichen planus.

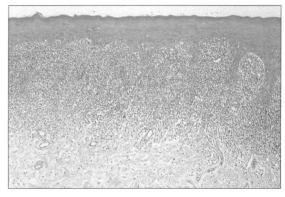

9.9 Lichen planus.

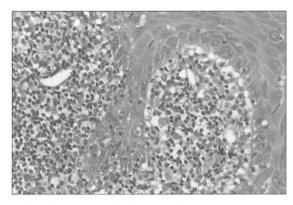

9.10 Lichen planus with Civatte bodies.

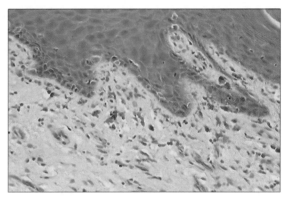

9.11 Lichen planus — pigmentary incontinence.

LUPUS ERYTHEMATOSUS

It can be difficult to distinguish lichen planus from lupus erythematosus. Lupus erythematosus, a multisystem disease, is associated with autoantibodies directed against DNA. In this specimen the epithelium is hyperkeratotic, and there is irregular downgrowth of the epithelium together with areas of epithelial atrophy (**9.12**). There is a distinctly thickened basement membrane zone and moderate atypia which in some lesions can occasionally simulate malignancy. Areas of Civatte body formation can also be seen (**9.13**). The inflammatory infiltrate is lymphohistiocytic and band-like in the superficial corium and extends in an irregular manner round some of the blood vessels. Patchy perivascular inflammatory infiltrate also occurs in the deeper tissues.

Oral lupus erythematosus may also show 'follicular plugging', which is the equivalent of keratin accumulation in the adnexal structures of the skin.

MUCOUS MEMBRANE PEMPHIGOID

This is a chronic immunologically mediated disease which affects the oral mucosa and can involve the eyes. In the mouth it forms bullae or manifests as desquamative gingivitis. Microscopy shows clean separation of the full thickness of the epithelium at the epithelio-mesenchymal junction. There is usually heavy chronic inflammation in the underlying connective tissue (**9.14**). As in pemphigus, the Nikolsky sign is positive and the epithelium may completely separate during the biopsy and be lost. The specimen then consists of non-specifically inflamed connective tissue which lacks a surface covering of fibrin slough that would be present if it were merely an ulcer. The diagnosis can be confirmed in frozen sections by direct immunofluorescence showing IgG (40% cases) or C3 (80% cases) deposition in the basement membrane zone (**9.15**). Indirect immunofluorescence (using the patient's serum) is frequently negative.

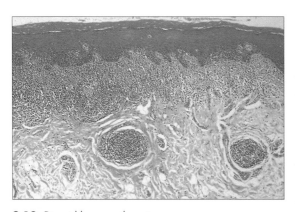

9.12 Discoid lupus erythematosus.

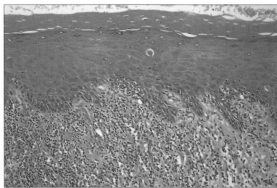

9.13 Discoid lupus erythematosus.

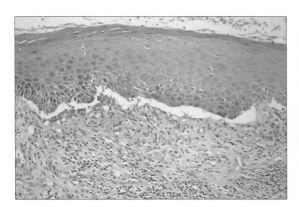

9.14 Mucous membrane pemphigoid.

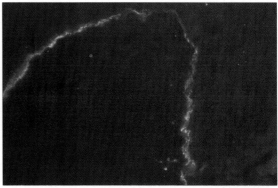

9.15 Mucous membrane pemphigoid — immunofluorescence staining IgG at the epithelio-mesenchymal junction.

ERYTHEMA MULTIFORME

Erythema multiforme affects stratified squamous epithelia and appears to be a hypersensitivity-type reaction to drugs, micro-organisms or other factors. As the name implies, the histology of erythema multiforme is extremely variable, but the most typical features are the formation of intraepithelial blisters mainly due to areas of intercellular oedema which coalesce to form vesicles (**9.16**). Occasionally eosinophilic coagulae develop within the upper part of the epithelium forming large, round eosinophilic bodies which are fibrinous in nature. There is a variable inflammatory reaction in the corium, sometimes with subepithelial vesiculation, particularly in the papillary corium (**9.17**). The inflammatory infiltrate seen depends to a large extent on the stage of the disease at which the biopsy is performed.

Later lesions show perivascular cuffing and sometimes frank vasculitis, and the whole of the epithelium becomes necrotic and sloughs. When an extensive inflammatory overlay exists the microscopical interpretation is difficult and may be entirely non-specific.

GEOGRAPHICAL TONGUE (ERYTHEMA MIGRANS)

Geographical tongue is a common idiopathic condition in which migrating areas of depapillation are seen on the dorsum of the tongue. Geographical tongue is infrequently biopsied, but has a very typical histological appearance. There is usually loss of the filiform papillae and a variable, although often minimal, inflammatory infiltrate in the corium. The most striking feature is the presence of polymorphs, usually in the upper part of the stratum spinosum (**9.18**). These may be scattered or aggregated into microabscesses when they are called spongiform pustules. These are not pathognomonic of geographical tongue and may be seen in several other oral conditions such as psoriasis (when they form microabscesses of Munro), candidosis (both acute and chronic), Reiter's syndrome and plasma cell gingivitis. There may be a psoriatic form of hyperplasia in geographical tongue and it may be impossible to distinguish the two conditions in the absence of a clinical history. Many pathologists believe that geographical tongue is the oral homology of psoriasis, but others will not accept a diagnosis of oral psoria-

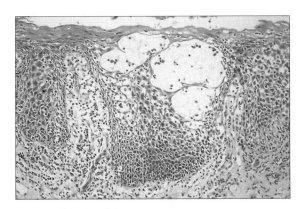

9.16 Erythema multiforme.

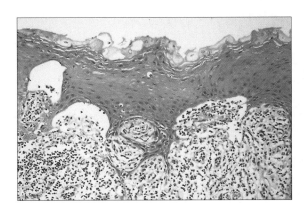

9.17 Erythema mutiforme.

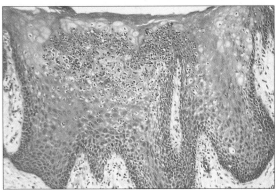

9.18 Geographical tongue.

sis in the absence of obvious and often severe cutaneous disease. Whenever spongiform pustules are seen in the upper epithelium it is important to search for candidal hyphae, because this is one of the most common causes of this type of appearance. Chronic candidosis can also result in a psoriatic form of hyperplasia. Typically, a much more florid inflammatory infiltrate is seen in the connective tissue, often with extensive fibrin leakage, and flakey surface parakeratosis. It is thus important to stain for candidal hyphae, either with the PAS stain or with a silver stain such as Grocott. The hyphae become more conspicuous and can be seen more readily by lowering the condenser which makes them more refractile. These hyphae are very easily overlooked and are readily missed by many non-specialist pathologists.

Identical features to geographical tongue can exist in other parts of the mouth, when they are called ectopic geographical tongue (but more appropriately, geographical stomatitis or migratory stomatitis). Similar lesions can be seen in Reiter's syndrome, and the differentiation is then based on clinical rather than histological features.

NON-SPECIFIC ULCERATION

Ulceration is the loss of surface epithelium. This slide shows a low-power view of an ulcer (**9.19**). The surface is covered by a mass of fibrin with intermingled, dead and dying polymorphs which would dry on the skin to form a crust or scab. However, in the mouth, which is continually moist, they form a slough which covers the floor of the ulcer. It is important to examine the surface of ulcers because it is possible for the epithelium to be lost by subepithelial vesiculation in conditions such as mucous membrane pemphigoid. In these circumstances, there is typically no evidence of surface slough because the specimen retained its epithelium until immediately before the biopsy. Therefore, a superficial ulcer with no evidence of significant fibrinous exudation on the surface or polymorph emigration suggests the possibility of a bullous disorder, particularly if there are clinical indications. A very heavy inflammatory infiltrate extends deep into the underlying connective tissue and blood vessels may show slight inflammatory vasculitis. There is granulation tissue formation with dilated blood vessels and a heavy infiltrate of plasma cells, lymphocytes and polymorphs.

9.19 Non-specific superficial ulcer.

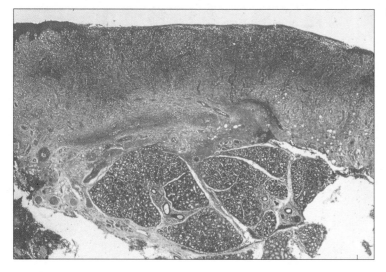

BEHÇET'S SYNDROME

Behçet's syndrome, although a multisystem disease which can affect many tissues, is an idiopathic condition characterised by recurrent aphthous stomatitis, often with genital ulcers and ocular lesions. This slide is from a cutaneous ulcer in Behçet's syndrome (**9.20**). There has been a considerable loss of tissue, depressing the ulcer well below the surface, and the inflammation extends deeply into the subcutaneous fat. The surface of the ulcer is covered by a fibrinous exudate infiltrated by polymorphs, which in this particular situation is forming a scab. A layer of granulation tissue with dilated capillaries and oedema is seen below (**9.21**). A repair reaction occurs below these features with fibrous tissue being laid down by the fibroblasts in the surrounding connective tissue, and a reduction in the amount of inflammation.

Some blood vessels show extensive fibrous proliferation of the subendothelial (intimal) connective tissue (**9.22**). This is an example of endarteritis obliterans, a non-specific feature which may be regarded as a protective response.

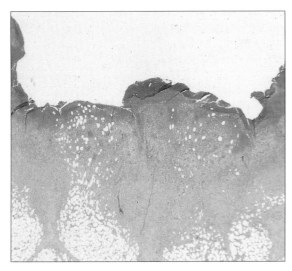

9.20 Behçet's syndrome — cutaneous ulcer.

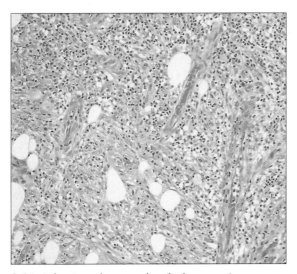

9.21 Behçet's syndrome — ulcer (higher power).

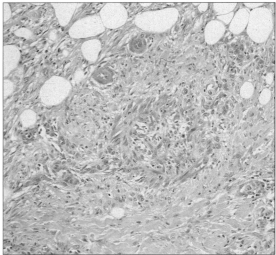

9.22 Behçet's syndrome — ulcer (higher power).

10.
WHITE PATCHES

WHITE SPONGE NAEVUS

White sponge naevi are inherited as an autosomal dominant trait and may be congenital or develop later in life. They characteristically produce thick, white plaques which can involve most of the oral mucosa. Microscopy shows shaggy parakeratosis and acanthosis with hydropic degeneration in the stratum spinosum (**10.1, 10.2**). There is usually no inflammatory component. Similar lesions may be present in the vagina or anus.

FRICTIONAL KERATOSIS

Frictional keratosis is a common cause of intraoral white patches and may be due to sharp edges of teeth or restorations or to cheek or lip chewing or sucking. It also commonly appears on the crest of the edentulous alveolus. Microscopy may show acanthosis or epithelial atrophy. There is a thick layer of orthokeratin and a prominent granular cell layer (**10.3, 10.4**). Less commonly there is hyperparakeratosis with absence of the granular cell layer. There is no dysplasia but there may be inflammation of the underlying corium, particularly if the area has ulcerated.

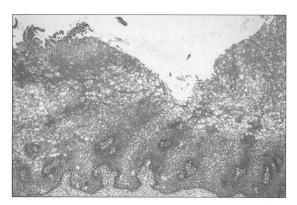

10.1 White sponge naevus.

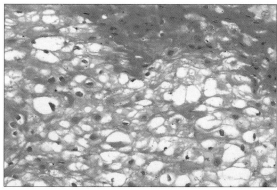

10.2 White sponge naevus (higher power).

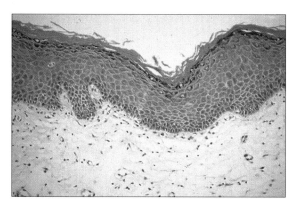

10.3 Frictional keratosis.

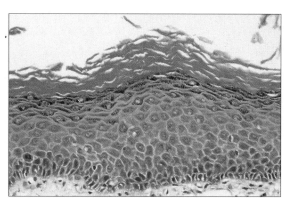

10.4 Frictional keratosis (higher power).

SMOKING RELATED KERATOSIS AND MELANOSIS

Smoking can result in intraoral plaque formation which clinically has a slatey blue colour. This specimen from the floor of the mouth has atrophic and hyperkeratotic epithelium, with patchy inflammation and melanin pigment in the underlying corium. There is no significant dysplasia (**10.5**). There has been pigmentary incontinence (release of melanin from damaged cells) and the melanin has been ingested by macrophages (melanophages) in the corium. Staining with Masson Fontana strikingly reveals melanin in the basal keratinocytes and the melanophages (**10.6**).

ACUTE CANDIDOSIS (THRUSH)

Acute candidosis forms creamy white plaques which can be rubbed off to leave a dry, red sore area of mucosa. Microscopy shows a loose parakeratotic plaque infiltrated by polymorphs and intraepithelial microabscesses (spongiform pustules) (see geographical tongue). The hyphae are difficult to see in haematoxylin and eosin stained sections but are readily visualised by staining with periodic acid Schiff (PAS) (**10.7**) or a silver stain such as Grocott's. There is variable, but occasionally florid, acute inflammation in the underlying corium.

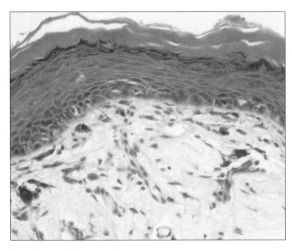

10.5 Smoker's keratosis.

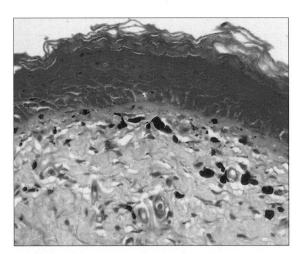

10.6 Smoker's keratosis. Masson Fontana stain.

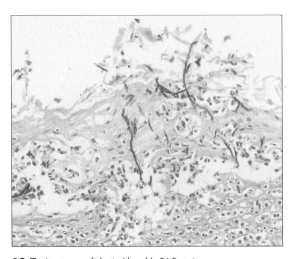

10.7 Acute candidosis (thrush). PAS stain.

CHRONIC HYPERPLASTIC CANDIDOSIS (CANDIDAL LEUKOPLAKIA)

Candida albicans may be present in persistent, adherent, firm white plaques which may be solitary or multiple, particularly in mucocutaneous candidosis syndromes. Microscopy shows a parakeratotic plaque infiltrated by polymorphs, spongiform pustules and acanthosis with inflammatory infiltration of the corium. The epithelium shows downgrowths of blunt or club-shaped rete ridges with thinning of the suprapapillary epithelium giving a resemblance to cutaneous psoriasis (so-called psoriasiform hyperplasia). The basement membrane zone may be thick and prominent and there is variable, but often severe, inflammation in the corium. In some cases there may be conspicuous fibrinous exudation, particularly in the papillary corium (**10.8**). As mentioned above, candidal hyphae may not be easily seen with haematoxylin and eosin stain but are readily visualised using the PAS technique.

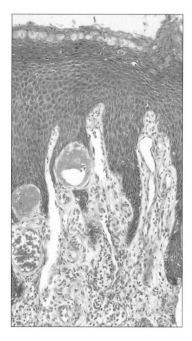

10.8 Chronic hyperplastic candidosis (candidal leukoplakia).

ORAL SUBMUCOUS FIBROSIS

Submucous fibrosis is virtually confined to Indian and Pakistani individuals. The oral mucosa becomes densely fibrosed so that opening becomes progressively impaired. Microscopy shows fibrosis of the connective tissue, atrophy of underlying muscle and the appearance of coarse, irregular elastic tissue (**10.9, 10.10**). Eventually the corium consists of hyalinised, relatively avascular scar tissue with patchy mononuclear infiltration. The overlying epithelium *eventually* shows atrophy and may become dysplastic.

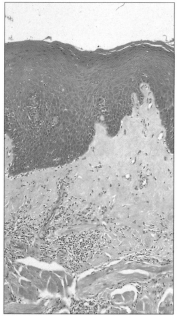

10.10 Submucous fibrosis (higher power).

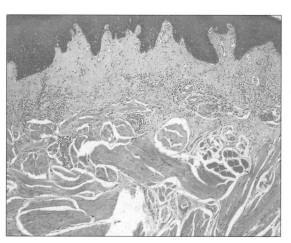

10.9 Submucous fibrosis.

HAIRY LEUKOPLAKIA

Patients infected with HIV frequently develop painless, corrugated (hairy) white plaques on the lateral border of the tongue and occasionally elsewhere in the mouth. Microscopy shows irregular parakeratosis, with or without candidal hyphae, and vacuolated cells with dark pyknotic nuclei (koilocytes) in the stratum spinosum (**10.11**). Even when candidal hyphae are present (**10.12**) there is usually no inflammatory infiltration of the epithelium (as in typical candidosis) or the underlying connective tissue. Immunocytochemical staining for Epstein–Barr capsid antigen in the epithelial nuclei is positive.

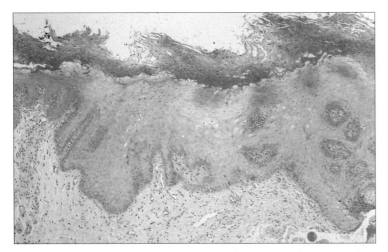

10.11 Hairy leukoplakia.

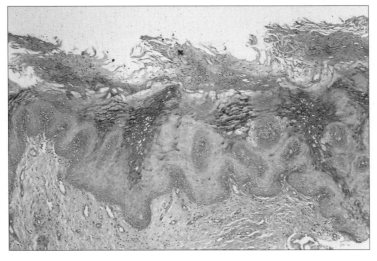

10.12 Hairy leukoplakia. PAS stain.

11.

PIGMENTED LESIONS

NORMAL MUCOSA

During embryological development, the skin and oral mucosa initially consist of keratinocytes while other cells, particularly melanocytes, appear later. The melanocytes are of neural crest origin, migrating through the corium to the basal cell layer of the epithelium. Ultimately, a ratio of approximately one melanocyte to every 10 basal keratinocytes is obtained. This forms what is known as an epidermal (epithelial) melanocyte unit. By light microscopy, melanocytes appear as clear cells in the basal layer. The nucleus and most of the cell have shrunk against the edge of what looks like a clear space (**11.1**). Stained with an appropriate stain such as Masson

Fontana the cells are seen to be dendritic. They produce melanin in preformed organelles called melanosomes, and then, by an as yet uncharacterised mechanism, they inject the melanosomes into the adjacent keratinocytes. As the basal keratinocytes divide and migrate up through the epithelial columns, the melanin is diluted into the surface layers.

MELANOTIC MACULES

The simplest type of pigmented lesion arising from melanocytes is when there is excess pigment formation in a focal area, i.e. a freckle (ephelis). Freckles result from localised areas of overactive melanocytes and heavily pigmented keratinocytes. In the oral mucosa these lesions are called melanotic macules. In addition to increased activity of basal melanocytes, pigmentary incontinence often occurs (**11.2**). The increased melanin in the basal keratinocytes, the melanin in the macrophages and the melanocytes themselves (which are dendritic) can be readily visualised using Masson Fontana stain (**11.3**).

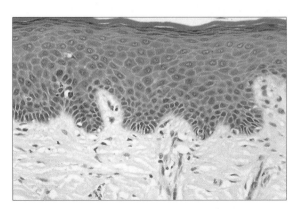

11.1 Melanocytes in basal layer of epithelium.

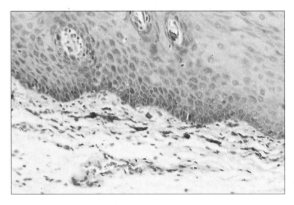

11.2 Melanotic macule.

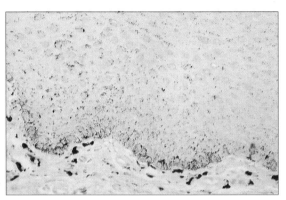

11.3 Melanotic macule. Masson Fontana stain.

RACIAL PIGMENTATION

Racial pigmentation is histologically similar to the melanotic macule. The increased pigmentation is due to increased synthesis of melanin by melanocytes which are otherwise normal in number and distribution (**11.4**).

NAEVI

Most children are born without cutaneous pigmented naevi (moles) which normally start to appear at about 12–18 months of age. Melanocytes proliferate at the epitheliomesenchymal junction in foci and frequently form nests. This is termed junctional activity and, if this is the only feature, the lesion is called a junctional naevus (**11.5**). Usually, however, nests of

cells 'drop off' into the underlying connective tissue where they form collections of naevus cells aggregated into discrete packets or theques (**11.6**). Naevus cells in the papillary corium may show some pigment production but those in the deeper corium are synthetically inactive. Lesions showing both junctional activity and naevus cells are called compound naevi.

Junctional activity usually ceases around the time of puberty. In pigmented naevi a normal ratio of melanocytes to basal cells overlying clumps of naevus cells results. In the skin this is termed an intradermal naevus and in the mouth an intramucosal naevus (**11.7**). There is usually no activity in the naevus cells. These cells usually contain little pigment but pigment-containing macrophages may be present. Naevus cells are typically aggregated into small groups and some may be multinucleated. The

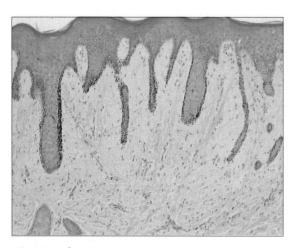

11.4 Racial pigmentation.

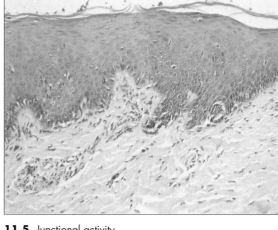

11.5 Junctional activity.

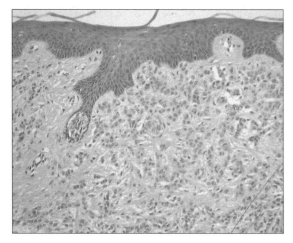

11.6 Compound naevus.

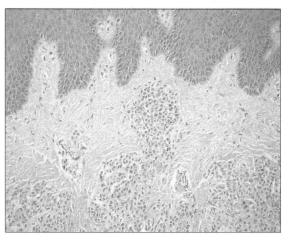

11.7 Intramucosal naevus.

naevus cells can be readily visualised with S100 stain (**11.8**). When a naevus matures, it tends to fibrose, particularly on the deeper aspect, and sometimes develops a striking resemblance to nerve tissue. This is then called a neuroid naevus (**11.9**). Fibrosis sometimes develops in the skin in relation to a naevus around a pilo-sebaceous unit. This can result in retrograde infection and abscess formation. Clinically the pigmented lesion suddenly increases in size, becomes painful and ulcerates, thus simulating malignancy. This phenomenon is not seen in oral lesions.

BLUE NAEVUS

The blue naevus is a relatively common type of intra-oral pigmented naevus. It forms from melanocytes which, during migration from the neural crest, become arrested below the basal cell layer to form a discrete tumour-like mass (**11.10**). Typically there is a focal collection of spindle-shaped cells which contain variable amounts of melanin. Usually there is a distinct gap between the overlying epithelium and the blue naevus. The naevus cells can be stained with S100 antibody or a melanin stain such as Masson Fontana (**11.11**).

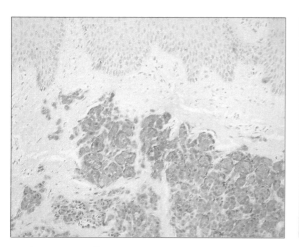

11.8 Intramucosal naevus. S100 stain.

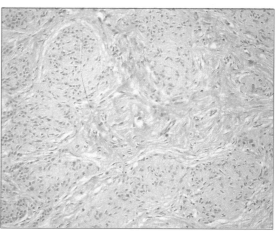

11.9 Neuroid naevus.

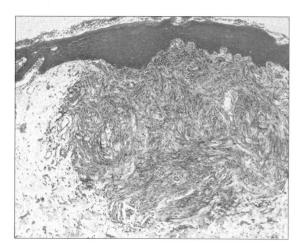

11.10 Blue naevus.

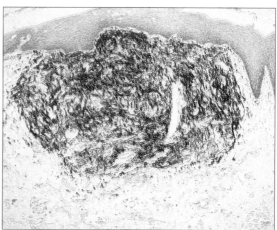

11.11 Blue naevus. Masson Fontana stain.

MELANOMA

In (malignant) melanoma there is a proliferation of melanocytes which are frankly abnormal and show cytological features of malignancy such as hyperchromatism, a high-nuclear cytoplasmic ratio and increased mitotic activity. There are degrees of invasion. In some melanomas the cells tend to invade through and along the epithelium as superficially spreading melanomas with a radial growth phase (**11.12**). In superficially spreading melanomas, downward invasion and nodule formation eventually ensues, rendering the lesion much more dangerous. Indeed, the prognosis of cutaneous melanomas is directly related to the thickness of the tumour (Breslow thickness). Most oral melanomas are nodular by the time they are discovered because they are usually symptomless in the earlier radial growth phase.

Melanomas have a variety of histological appearances. In the example shown the cells are rather spindle-shaped (**11.13**). Typically there is no inflammatory infiltrate in relation to benign pigmented lesions — the presence of which is always slightly alarming. The pigmentation in melanomas is very variable and may be found in tumour cells or macrophages (**11.14**). In some tumours no melanin can be found (amelanotic melanoma). Epithelial hyperplasia, another feature which is not uncommon, may be striking (**11.15**). The important differential diagnosis is therefore spindle cell squamous carcinoma although patchy melanotic pigmentation can be seen in the spindle-shaped cells at high power (**11.16**).

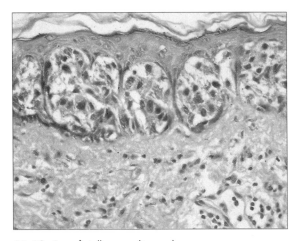

11.12 Superficially spreading melanoma.

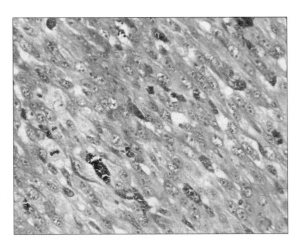

11.13 Melanoma.

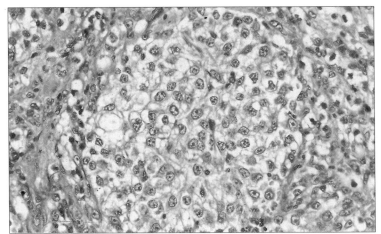

11.14 Melanoma.

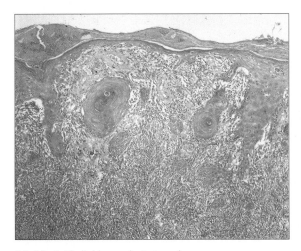

11.15 Epithelial hyperplasia in melanoma.

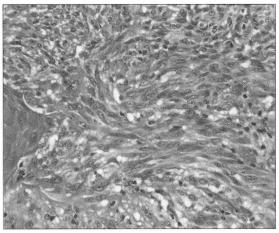

11.16 Spindle-shaped melanoma cells below area of epithelial hyperplasia (higher power).

PIGMENTED NEUROECTODERMAL TUMOUR OF INFANCY

Pigmented neuroectodermal tumours are usually seen within the first two or three months of life as destructive lesions, typically in the anterior maxilla although they have also been reported in other parts of the head and neck. They tend to resolve with minimal treatment.

Pigmented neuroectodermal tumours consist of two cell types: pigmented melanin-containing cells which are small, dark and either form clumps or cleft-like spaces, and clear cells, with no pigment, which either form separate islands or lie within clefts lined by pigmented cells (**11.17, 11.18**). There is a non-inflamed, fibroblastic stroma. These tumours appear to be neuroectodermal in origin and may produce excess secretion of catecholamines, detectable by assay of urinary metabolites.

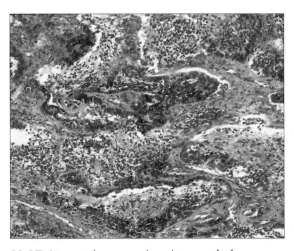

11.17 Pigmented neuroectodermal tumour of infancy.

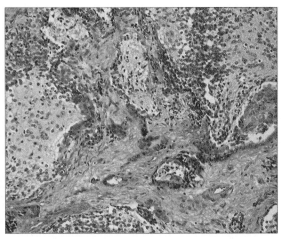

11.18 Pigmented neuroectodermal tumour of infancy.

AMALGAM TATTOOS

Amalgam tattoos are probably the most common localised pigmented lesions in the mouth and usually result from mucosal abrasions obtained during a dental restorative procedure. Microscopy shows black amalgam pigment either in lumps (**11.19**) or finely dispersed along collagen bundles and around blood vessels and nerves (causing similar staining as a silver histological stain) (**11.20**). Inflammation is variable and occasionally there is a granulomatous reaction to the amalgam with foreign-body multi-nucleated giant cells.

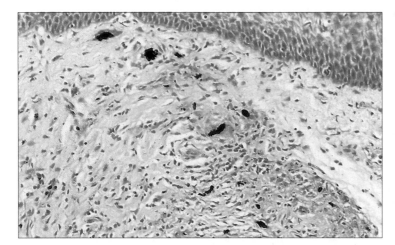

11.19 Amalgam tattoo.

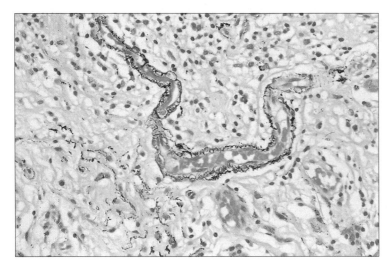

11.20 Amalgam tattoo.

12.

SOFT TISSUE SWELLINGS

FIBROEPITHELIAL POLYPS

Fibroepithelial polyps, or fibrous overgrowths, are the most common intraoral lumps and may be sessile or pedunculated. Microscopically they consist of a core of fibrous tissue of variable cellularity and an overlying epithelium which may be normal, hyperplastic and often hyperkeratinised (either parakeratinised or orthokeratinised) (**12.1**). Sometimes fibroepithelial polyps are rich in mucopolysaccharides and have a bluish hue on haematoxylin and eosin staining. Polyps may ulcerate if they impinge on an adjacent structure such as a tooth or a denture. Unless they are ulcerated there is usually little inflammation.

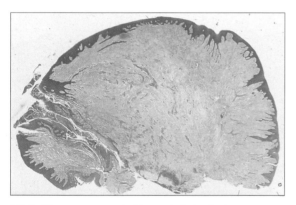

12.1 Fibrous overgrowth (fibroepithelial polyp).

GIANT CELL FIBROMAS

Giant cell fibromas are most frequently seen on the gingiva and tongue, usually as pedunculated polyps. They contain multinucleated fibroblasts in a heavily collagenised core. The fibroblasts are typically triangular or stellate and often have double or multiple nuclei, but they are not typical giant cells (**12.2**). The fibroblasts close to the surface epithelium may contain melanin.

FIBROUS EPULIDES

Fibrous epulides are common gingival lumps. Like other fibrous overgrowths, they show variable degrees of cellularity and collagenisation. Typically the epithelium is either normal or hyperplastic, below which is an area of fibroblastic proliferation and collagenisation, sometimes with dense inflammation.

In the fibrous epulis shown, there is an ulcerated hyperplastic epithelium producing an acutely inflamed surface (**12.3**). The bulk of the lesion consists of a vascular stroma with plump fibroblasts showing large vesicular nuclei and prominent nucleoli. There may be mitotic activity which can be somewhat alarming at higher power (**12.4**). Dystrophic calcification, due to the deposition of

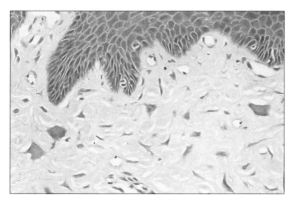

12.2 Giant cell fibroma.

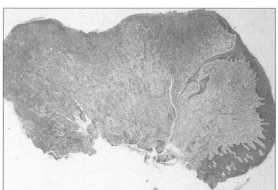

12.3 Fibrous epulis.

calcium salts around non-vital tissues, is common in both fibrous and giant cell epulides. In fibrous epulides, osseous metaplasia is common and may be extensive (**12.5**). Conservative excision is usually curative but lesions sometimes recur, occasionally several times.

GIANT CELL EPULIDES

The giant cell epulis usually forms a fleshy bluish swelling on the gingiva, most frequently anterior to the first molars. Histologically there is usually a cell-free zone between the main lesion and the overlying epithelium but this tends to be lost if there is inflammation or ulceration (**12.6**). There is a matrix or stroma of plump spindle-shaped cells which are interspersed with multinucleated giant cells. These are sometimes so confluent that it can be difficult to see the outlines of the giant cells. The cells are large and contain about 10–20 nuclei. There are two main giant cell types: one in which the cytoplasm is lightly eosinophilic and the nuclei are large, vesicular and have prominent nucleoli, and the other type which has a much more densely stained cytoplasm with pyknotic and densely haematoxyphilic nuclei (**12.7**). The latter probably results from degeneration of the first type. The giant cell epulis can be extremely vascular and sometimes shows multinucleated giant cells within the vascular spaces (**12.7**). There may be considerable amounts of haemosiderin in these lesions. Mitotic activity is usually not difficult to find, but bears no relation to the clinical behaviour. Osseous metaplasia is common and sometimes florid. Giant cell epulides tend to recur after excision.

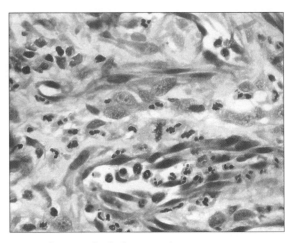

12.4 Fibrous epulis (higher power).

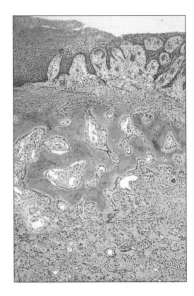

12.5 Fibrous epulis with osseous metaplasia.

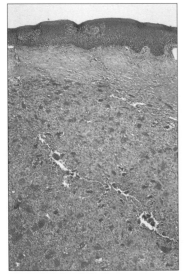

12.6 Giant cell epulis.

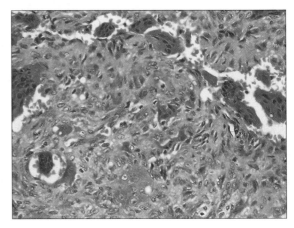

12.7 Giant cell epulis (higher power).

FIBROSARCOMAS

True fibromas are extremely uncommon and are among the least frequent of all tumours, despite the fact that fibrous tissue is the most ubiquitous of all tissues.

Although fibrosarcomas are much more common, they are still rare within the mouth. Fibrosarcomas are spindle-cell tumours, often forming interweaving fasciculae and a so-called herring bone configuration (**12.8**). The cells show moderate degrees of pleomorphism. There is a high mitotic rate in some examples (**12.9**). It is not uncommon to find multinucleated tumour cells, particularly in the less well-differentiated tumours. Some fibrosarcomas are difficult to distinguish histologically from other tumours such as malignant fibrous histiocytoma and leiomyosarcoma, but the behaviour of these tumours is similar.

AMPUTATION NEUROMAS

Special stains are often unhelpful in diagnostic pathology but the example shown illustrates the use of an immunocytochemical stain, S100, which simplifies diagnosis. The haematoxylin and eosin stain shows a non-descript mass of moderately cellular fibrous tissue (**12.10**) while the S100 stain shows a tangled mass of proliferating nerve fibres typical of an amputation (traumatic) neuroma (**12.11**).

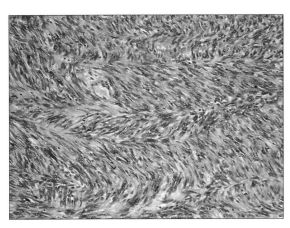

12.8 Fibrosarcoma.

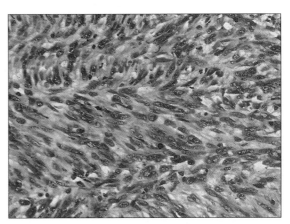

12.9 Fibrosarcoma (higher power).

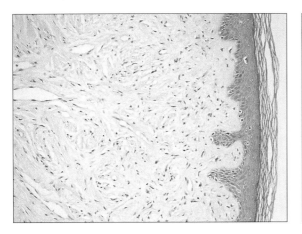

12.10 Amputation neuroma.

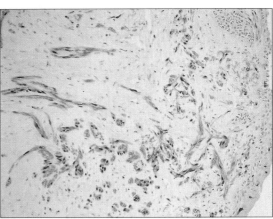

12.11 Amputation neuroma. S100 stain.

NEUROFIBROMAS

The neurofibroma is a discrete, but usually non-encapsulated, mass of spindle-shaped cells (**12.12**) which may show slight interfasciculation. Many of the spindle-shaped cells stain for S100 (**12.13**). In some areas, they show a tendency to aggregate as sinuous bands and give an appearance reminiscent of a true nerve structure. Neurofibromas are often closely juxtaposed to a nerve. Another common feature of neurofibromas is the presence of many mast cells (**12.14**).

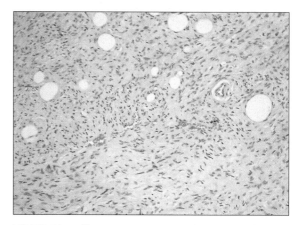

12.12 Neurofibroma.

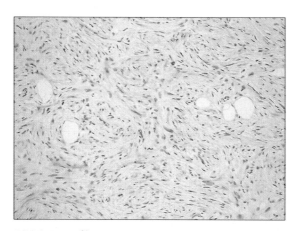

12.13 Neurofibroma. S100 stain.

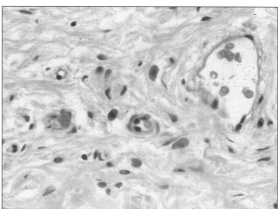

12.14 Neurofibroma showing mast cells.

NEURILEMMOMAS

Neurilemmomas are typically quite large encapsulated tumours and consist of two main types of tissue which vary considerably in proportion within any particular tumour. Antoni A tissue consists of spindle-shaped cells forming an interwoven pattern — areas of which may show palisaded or regimented nuclei (**12.15**). The nuclei may aggregate into organoid structures called Verocay bodies. Antoni B tissue is a rather myxoid element (**12.16**). As in neurofibromas, mast cells may be plentiful. Not infrequently there is a tendency for the Antoni B tissue to degenerate and occasionally become hyalinised and fibrosed, particularly in long-standing neurilemmomas (which are then called ancient neurilemmomas). This is an important variant, because the cells in the degenerating area can appear pleomorphic and simulate malignancy.

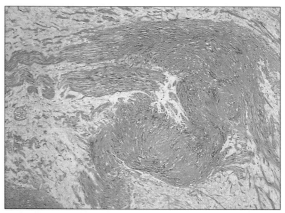

12.15 Neurilemmoma.

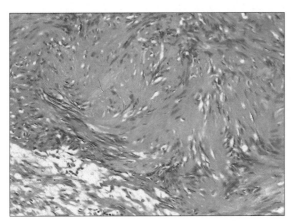

12.16 Neurilemmoma (higher power).

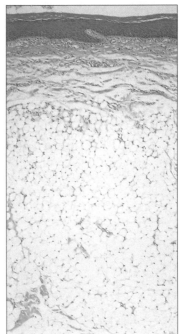

12.17 Lipoma.

LIPOMAS

Oral lipomas are moderately common. They usually present as either a sessile or pedunculated yellowish nodule, commonly in the buccal mucosa or on the tongue.

Microscopically, lipomas consist of a well circumscribed mass of mature fat cells with no capsule (**12.17**). The only feature of note is the presence of cells with vacuolated nuclei, called Lochkern cells (**12.18**). These cells are also seen in mature fat but are of no other significance. Sometimes focal collections of vacuolated cells are present within lipomas. These are macrophages which have ingested fat, and are termed lipophages. Occasionally prominent vascular elements develop within the tumour, which some pathologists then term an 'angiolipoma'. If there is associated fibrous connective tissue, which may be hyalinised, the tumour is called a fibrolipoma (**12.19**).

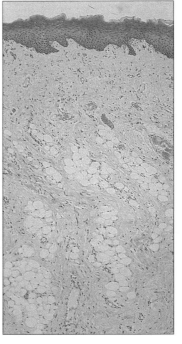

12.19 Fibrolipoma.

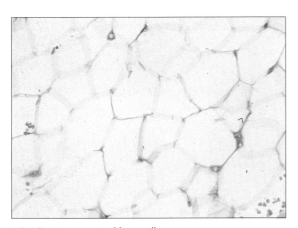

12.18 Lipoma — Lochkern cells.

RHABDOMYOMAS

The rhabdomyoma is an uncommon tumour in any site, but is virtually restricted to the head and neck region. It usually presents as a discrete rubbery swelling, often in the floor of the mouth when it can resemble a sublingual dermoid.

Rhabdomyomas have a characteristic appearance at low power microscopy . The cells are granular, circumscribed and very pink on haematoxylin and eosin staining and have many small spaces which superficially makes the lesion resemble a fatty tumour. The vacuolated spaces are filled with intracytoplasmic glycogen which is lost during processing (**12.20**).

Sometimes intracytoplasmic crystalloid material may also be seen. Most of the cells are rounded or strap-shaped and some have a rather spider-web appearance as the cytoplasm tends to shrink away from the cell membrane. These cells are immature striated muscle cells. Although this is a tumour of striated muscle it is often difficult to see the striations. The best place to observe the cross-striations is in the strap-shaped cells at the periphery. This type of tumour often requires special staining, such as phosphotungstic acid haematoxylin (PTAH) staining, which enhances the cross-striations for confirmation of diagnosis (**12.21**).

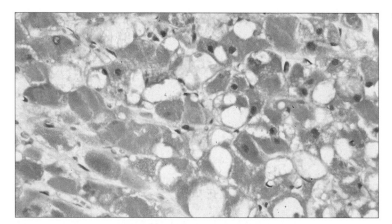

12.20 Rhabdomyoma.

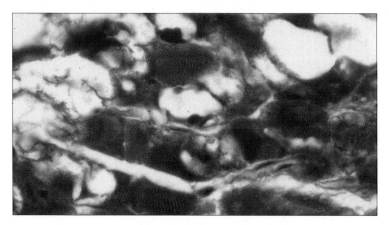

12.21 Rhabdomyoma. PTAH stain.

RHABDOMYOSARCOMAS

Rhabdomyosarcomas are much more common than rhabdomyomas and exist as several different types. The most common is an **embryonal rhabdomyosarcoma**, typically seen in infants and children, which consists of immature malignant striated muscle cells (rhabdomyoblasts) showing variable degrees of pleomorphism. The embryonal rhabdomyosarcoma contains spindle-shaped cells with obvious features of malignancy such as gross pleomorphism, high mitotic activity and nuclear hyperchromatism (**12.22**). The diagnosis depends on the recognition of rhabdomyoblasts, which can be large cells varying in shape and size with pale eosinophilic cytoplasm. Rhabdomyoblasts may be strap-shaped, round or multinucleated (**12.23**). Cross-striations can be difficult to see with haematoxylin and eosin staining but can be visualised with PTAH stain. Sometimes the cells stain for myosin or myoglobin.

Embryonal rhabdomyosarcomas may also be seen on surfaces, typically the bladder, vagina and nasal cavity, when they produce grape-like excrescences and are known as botryoid rhabdomyosarcomas. A strong characteristic of this variant is a cell-free zone between the surface epithelium and the tumour, called the cambian layer (**12.24**).

The **alveolar rhabdomyosarcoma** is seen more typically in adolescents and sometimes older people, and is much more common in deep muscle tissue when the cells either form sheets or interweaving fascicles, which infiltrate muscle. It forms alveolar spaces (**12.25**) with thin, fibrous septa. The rhabdomyoblasts typically line or hang from the fibrous septa or float freely within the spaces. The rhab-

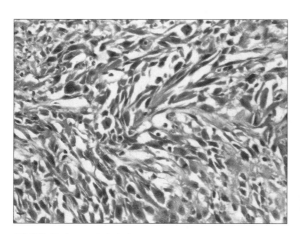

12.22 Embryonal rhabdomyosarcoma.

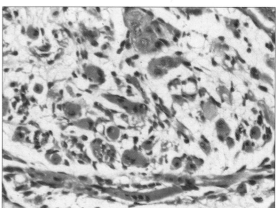

12.23 Embryonal rhabdomyosarcoma.

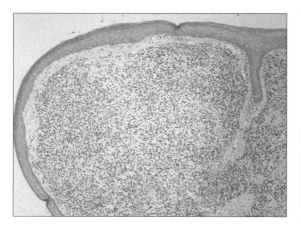

12.24 Embryonal rhabdomyosarcoma — botryoid variant.

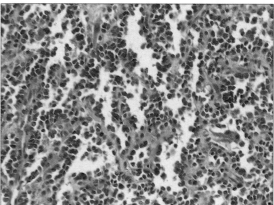

12.25 Alveolar rhabdomyosarcoma.

domyoblasts in this variant tend to be small and rounded and in solid areas can easily be confused with lymphocytes (**12.26**). Cross-striations may be very difficult to find.

The **pleomorphic rhabdomyosarcoma** is the other main type of rhabdomyosarcoma. This tends to be a spindle cell tumour with very little rhabdomyoblastic differentiation. There may be considerable difficulty in differentiating this from other spindle cell tumours and the diagnosis may be totally unsuspected because the lesion tends to arise in adolescents and adults rather than children. Pleomorphic rhabdomyosarcomas have many large pleomorphic cells, some of which are multinucleated (**12.27**). A high-power view shows gross pleomorphism and bizarre mitoses (**12.28**).

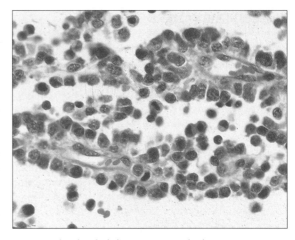

12.26 Alveolar rhabdomyosarcoma (higher power).

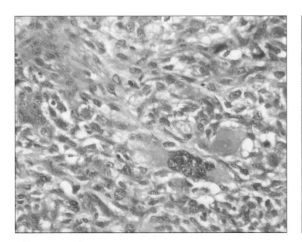

12.27 Pleomorphic rhabdomyosarcoma.

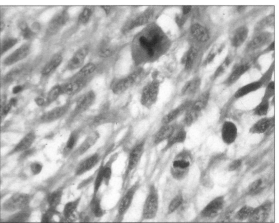

12.28 Pleomorphic rhabdomyosarcoma (higher power).

LEIOMYOMAS

Leiomyomas arise in the orofacial tissues from the smooth muscle of blood vessels and are therefore also termed angiomyomas (**12.29**). The smooth muscle cells, which do not show pleomorphism, are arranged around vascular lumina of variable sizes and often in a clearly recognisable vacular configuration.

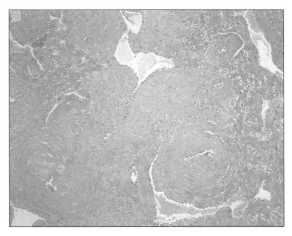

12.29 Angiomyoma (leiomyoma).

LEIOMYOSARCOMAS

Leiomyosarcomas are rare and are usually well-differentiated. The cells are arranged in interweaving fasciculae resulting in cells being cut in various planes (**12.30**). The characteristic feature of leiomyosarcomas is the nuclei (particularly in well-differentiated tumours) which are either cigar-shaped or have a blunt or sometimes even indented end (**12.31**). PTAH will help identify longitudinal filaments in the strap-shaped cells.

In some smooth muscle tumours it is difficult to decide whether the tumour is benign or malignant. However, almost any degree of mitotic activity in a smooth muscle tumour suggests malignancy.

CONGENITAL EPULIDES

The congenital epulis is usually seen in the newborn child as a sessile or pedunculated swelling, typically in the anterior maxilla. They are much more common in females with a ratio of 10:1. A congenital epulis will often protrude from the mouth as a reddish swelling.

The overlying epithelium is typically normal or attenuated and covers a circumscribed mass of pink, round, granular cells which are usually in a moderately vascular fibrous stroma (**12.32**). The cells have distinct cell membranes and are oncocytic and granular on haematoxylin and eosin staining; they show similarity to those seen in some granular cell tumours. The cell of origin is not known although some pathologists believe they are related to Schwann cells while others consider that they arise from undifferentiated mesenchymal cells. The lesion is entirely benign and conservative excision is curative.

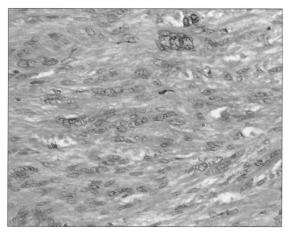

12.30 Leiomyosarcoma.

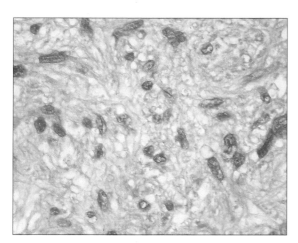

12.31 Leiomyosarcoma (higher power).

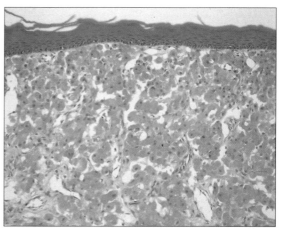

12.32 Congenital epulis.

GRANULAR CELL TUMOURS

Granular cell tumours (myoblastomas) are not uncommon tumours of the skin and mucosal surfaces. They arise particularly in the mouth, where the dorsum of the tongue is the typical site. The lesion usually presents as a non-descript slow-growing, painless lump which occasionally resembles a tumour macroscopically.

Unfortunately, this simulation can also be seen microscopically. This particular example shows very striking pseudoepitheliomatous hyperplasia of the overlying epithelium but inconspicuous granular cells (**12.33**). At low power, the lesion simulates a squamous cell carcinoma. However, between the underlying muscle and the epithelium are the granular cells that form the basis of the lesion. Granular cells tend to be round or strap-shaped, have coarse granules, and sometimes appear to fuse with normal muscle (**12.34**). These cells were once thought to originate from muscle cells giving rise to the term granular cell myoblastomas. However, despite the fact that the cells seem to fuse with the muscle, they appear to be of Schwann cell origin. The cells stain with S100 and neurone-specific enolase.

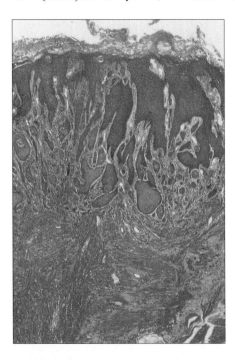

12.33 Granular cell tumour.

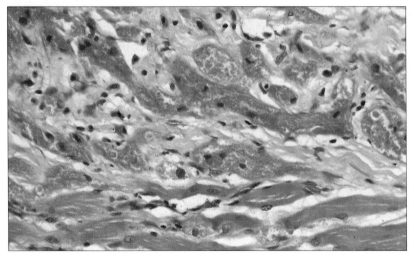

12.34 Granular cell tumour (higher power).

13.
LESIONS AFFECTING BLOOD VESSELS

GIANT CELL ARTERITIS

Formerly known as temporal or cranial arteritis, this disorder frequently affects the craniofacial arteries of elderly patients, particularly women, causing pain. The main importance of giant cell arteritis is the fact that the vessels involved may become occluded and if the central artery of the retina (which is an end artery) is affected, the patient becomes blind. It is, therefore, important that the condition is recognised clinically before there is any permanent damage. Giant cell arteritis may also form part of the more generalised condition of polymyalgia rheumatica.

The temporal artery is frequently affected and is the likely biopsy site. Microscopy shows an inflammatory reaction in the intima and media, with infiltration of lymphocytes, fragmentation of the elastic lamina and accumulation of multinucleated giant cells (**13.1**). In turn, there is extensive intimal proliferation producing obliterative endarteritis (**13.2**). Unfortunately, since the changes tend to be patchy, the biopsy can miss the area showing characteristic changes. From a practical point-of-view, the best course of action is to put the patient with suspected giant cell arteritis on a high dose of corticosteroids and to assay the erythrocyte sedimentation rate (ESR), plasma viscosity or C-reactive protein (CRP). If these are raised, this diagnosis is probably correct.

RADIATION DAMAGE

Following radiation exposure, the collagen in the lower part of the corium tends to show elastotic degeneration, which has a similar appearance to actinic-induced damage. The collagen becomes coarse and wavy and not only resembles elastic tissue but stains similarly. In addition, small arteries show endarteritis, with proliferation of the intima and luminal narrowing (**13.3**). There is very little change in the venules. Endarteritis may result in a compromised blood supply to the tissues and secondary ischaemic changes, with subsequent loss of adnexal structures in the irradiated skin or mucosa. Dilatation

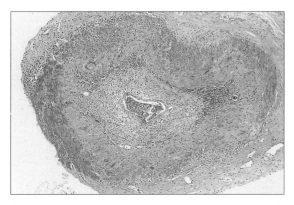

13.1 Giant cell arteritis.

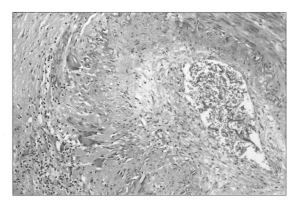

13.2 Giant cell arteritis (higher power).

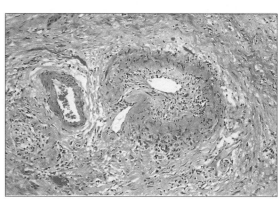

13.3 Radiation-induced endarteritis.

of the superficial capillaries may also produce telangiectasia (**13.4**). A very typical feature of irradiated skin or mucosa is the development of fibrosis, some of which is possibly secondary to ischaemia (in addition to the direct consequence of irradiation). Bizarre ('radiation') fibroblasts, which can be multinucleated, stellate or triangular in shape, can be seen within otherwise acellular tissue.

HAEMANGIOMAS

Haemangiomas are common. They are hamartomas, a type of growth disorder which typically tends to grow at the same rate as the rest of the body, often forming a tumour-like mass which usually stabilises when somatic growth ceases. Although many haemangiomas are congenital, some develop in later life.

The capillary-type of haemangioma consists of predominantly solid cores of endothelial cells with very small lumina, and prominent vessels (**13.5**). The lesion often extends into the underlying adnexal structures, such as minor salivary glands, and muscle. There is usually little or no evidence of mitotic activity and minimal inflammation unless the lesions have been traumatised. The two latter features can help differentiate a capillary haemangioma from a pyogenic granuloma or occasionally organising granulation tissue.

Cavernous haemangiomas are much more common in the mouth than capillary haemangiomas. They consist simply of an excessive number of dilated, thin-walled vessels, with or without evidence of previous haemorrhage (**13.6**). Sometimes trauma leads to interstitial haemorrhage or thrombosis which is then followed by organisation of the blood clot into fibrous-tissue. When this happens there can be a striking proliferation of endothelial cells, often forming papillary processes (papillary endothelial hyperplasia) which can simulate angiosarcoma.

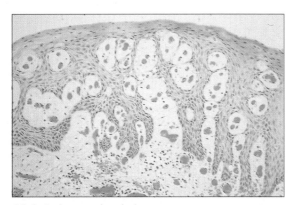

13.4 Radiation-induced telangiectasia.

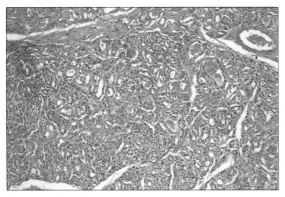

13.5 Capillary haemangioma.

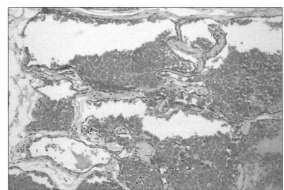

13.6 Cavernous haemangioma.

LYMPHANGIOMAS

Lymphangiomas either present as localised swellings within the mouth or as larger lesions in the neck (cystic hygromas). Intraoral lymphangiomas tend to form bosselated swellings which have a tendency to become blackened when there is interstitial haemorrhage into the lesion. This discolouration may be the patient's immediate complaint. Sometimes they are associated with gross malformation of the tongue (macroglossia) or lips (macrocheilia). Lymphangiomas consist of large dilated spaces which are either empty or filled with proteinaceous fluid (**13.7**). Haemorrhage into the spaces is common and occasionally the lesions may be difficult to differentiate from haemangiomas. However, lymphangiomas typically extend into the surface epithelium, which is why they appear granular and framboesiform clinically. It is also common to find an associated lymphocytic infiltrate which is not an inflammatory reaction but rather an integral part of the lesion (**13.8**).

KAPOSI'S SARCOMA

Kaposi's sarcoma is seen mainly in AIDS patients and presents as a macule or nodule, typically purple or brown, especially in the palate. In the initial stages of development, the lesion histologically resembles granulation tissue with dilated vascular spaces, proliferation of endothelial cells and fibroblasts (**13.9**). However, Kaposi's sarcoma differs from typical granulation tissue because there is minimal oedema and polymorph infiltration. As the lesions of Kaposi's sarcoma mature, they become more fibroblastic and spindle cell-like, so that superficially they can resemble a fibrosarcoma (**13.10**). Mitotic activity is present, but it is not particularly florid (more would be seen in a fibrosarcoma). Characteristic features of Kaposi's sarcoma include the vascularity and slit-like vascular spaces which contain red blood cells. There may be extravasation of red blood cells with haemosiderin deposition.

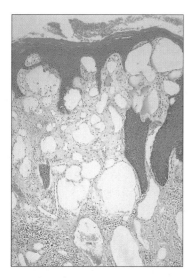

13.7 Lymphangioma.

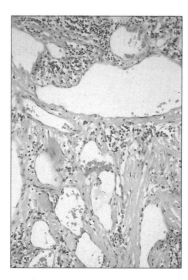

13.8 Lymphangioma (higher power).

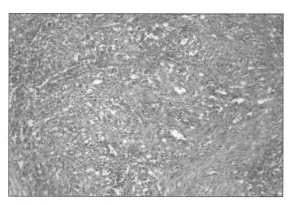

13.9 Kaposi's sarcoma.

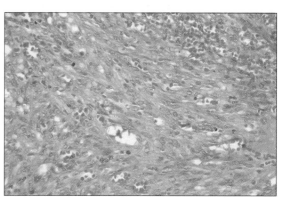

13.10 Kaposi's sarcoma.

EOSINOPHILIC ULCERS (TRAUMATIC EOSINOPHILIC GRANULOMAS)

Eosinophilic ulceration is uncommon and usually affects the tongue. It is predominantly associated with trauma, usually crush injury. Typically there is a deep ulcer which superficially shows non-specific histological features although there is a dense infiltrate of histiocytes and eosinophils in the deeper layers which extends into the underlying muscle (which may show evidence of damage). In some cases the histiocytes may show a brisk mitotic rate which, together with regenerating endothelial cells, can lead to a erroneous diagnosis of malignancy (**13.11**). There is no relationship between this lesion and the eosinophilic granuloma (Langerhan's cell histiocytosis).

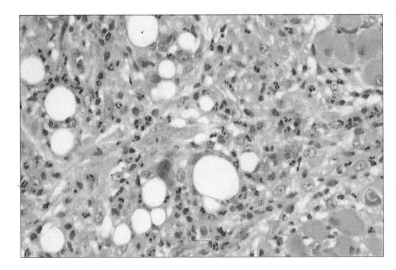

13.11 Eosinophilic ulcer.

14.
SQUAMOUS EPITHELIAL TUMOURS

SQUAMOUS PAPILLOMA

Squamous papillomas are usually small, sessile or pedunculated lesions which are not particularly common in the oral mucosa. They have a fibrovascular core, extensions of which are covered by acanthotic stratified squamous epithelium (**14.1**). The epithelium shows no evidence of dysplasia but there may be some koilocytic change — clear cells with the nucleus pushed to one side. It is probable that the majority of papillomas are viral in origin — koilocytosis is a feature of some viral infections. There is no tendency for malignant change.

PAPILLARY HYPERPLASIA

Papillary hyperplasia is seen in the vault of the palate as papillary excrescences, usually in the midline and frequently associated with denture-wearing.

Biopsy shows multiple fibrovascular cores and often very hyperplastic stratified squamous epithelium which grows down into the underlying connective tissue core. This appearance can simulate malignancy (**14.2**). Papillary hyperplasia is one of the oral pseudoepitheliomatous conditions. Usually there is no significant atypia in the downgrowths but often a moderate amount of chronic inflammation can be seen in the connective tissue. It is occasionally possible to see superimposed candidosis although this does not appear to be important in the pathogenesis.

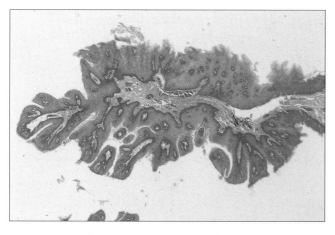

14.1 Squamous papilloma.

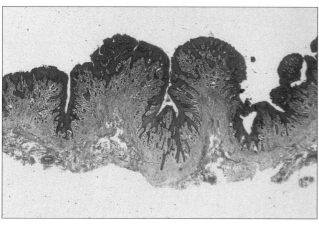

14.2 Papillary hyperplasia of the palate.

DYSPLASIA

Epithelial dysplasia (or atypia) is the collective histological term used to describe disordered cell maturation and proliferation associated with an increased risk of progression to malignancy. Pathologists make an essentially subjective judgement of the degree of dysplasia present based on varying combinations of a diverse range of histological features. These changes include:

(1) Irregular hyperplasia (increased cell numbers) particularly of cells with a basal cell morphology (basal cell hyperplasia). Epithelial atrophy, which may be clinically associated with erythroplasia, may sometimes be a feature of severe dysplasia.

(2) Rete ridges showing a drop-shaped configuration is also a feature of severe dysplasia.

(3) Loss of both polarity of cells and normal stratification of the epithelial layer.

(4) Nuclear changes such as an increased nuclear-cytoplasmic ratio, more intense nuclear staining (hyperchromatism) and variations in shape and size (pleomorphism).

(5) Mitoses in the upper levels of the epithelium, excess numbers or abnormal mitoses such as triradiate forms.

(6) Individual cell keratinisation often in the deep layers (dyskeratosis or premature keratinisation).

(7) Loss of intercellular cohesion giving a tendency for cells to separate and, in extreme cases, acantholysis (malignant acantholysis).

Mild degrees of dysplasia can be seen in non-neoplastic reactive lesions such as the regenerating epithelium at the edge of an ulcer, or overlying inflammatory lesions. Although dysplastic lesions can regress, the risk of progression to overt malignancy increases with the degree of dysplasia. The term 'carcinoma-*in-situ*' is used by some pathologists to describe dysplastic lesions when the abnormalities involve the whole thickness of the epithelium. This is uncommon in oral mucosa as even severe dysplasia tends to show some differentiation at the surface. Such lesions often present as idiopathic red patches (erythroplasia) or speckled leukoplakia.

These changes are illustrated in the following examples. **14.3** shows epithelial atrophy while the lower half of the epithelium consists of cells with a basal cell morphology and a high nuclear cytoplasmic ratio. There are conspicuous intercellular spaces (loss of cohesion) and an increased mitotic rate with some suprabasal mitoses. This is moderate dysplasia.

14.4 shows hyperplasia with some basal cell hyperplasia and hyperchromatism. There is excess mitotic activity and several suprabasal mitoses. This also illustrates moderate dysplasia.

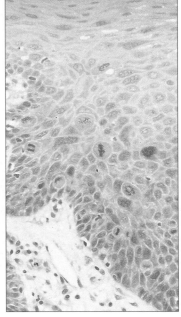

14.4 Moderate dysplasia.

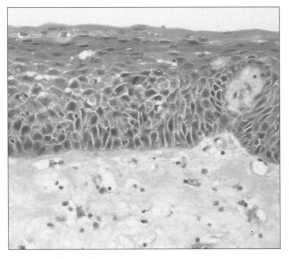

14.3 Moderate dysplasia.

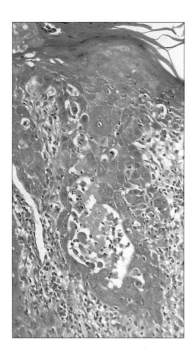

14.5 Moderate dysplasia.

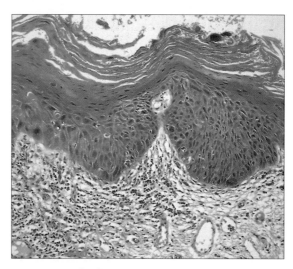

14.6 Severe dysplasia.

14.5 shows intercellular oedema, dyskeratosis and high level, excess mitotic activity. This indicates moderate dysplasia.

14.6 and **14.7** show drop-shaped rete ridges, loss of stratification, basal cell hyperplasia with pleomorphism, dyskeratosis, excess and high-level mitoses with changes extending throughout most of the thickness of the epithelium. This is severe dysplasia which some would consider to be carcinoma *in-situ*. Drop-shaped rete ridges are particularly associated with a high tendency towards malignant progression.

14.8 shows severe intercellular oedema (malignant acantholysis) in the lower half of the epithelium together with an excess number of mitoses (which are also high-level) and dyskeratosis. Although the changes only involve the lower part of the epithelium many pathologists would consider this to be severe dysplasia.

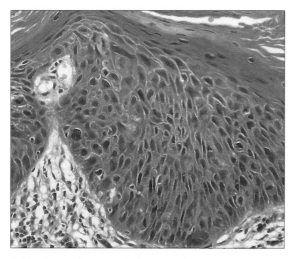

14.7 Severe dysplasia (higher power).

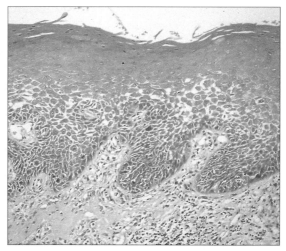

14.8 Malignant acantholysis in moderately severe dysplasia.

SQUAMOUS CELL CARCINOMA

Oral squamous cell carcinomas are most commonly found on the lateral margin of the tongue or floor of the mouth in older men. They may be associated with tobacco and alcohol use.

Oral squamous cell carcinomas mainly present as an ulcer, lump, or red or white lesion. Frankly invasive carcinomas often show a lower degree of dysplasia than some non-invasive dysplastic lesions. **14.9** shows a typical, well-differentiated squamous cell carcinoma. The epithelium is forming islands which resemble normal stratified squamous epithelium, except that they are invading the underlying tissues and undergoing aberrant keratinisation. Instead of the keratin being formed and shed from the surface, it is formed within the substance of an epithelial island producing a keratin whorl or epithelial pearl. This is a feature of well-differentiated carcinoma.

The epithelial islands may be discrete and circumscribed, even though they are invading the underlying tissues quite extensively, or appear more moth-eaten with loss of basement membrane (**14.10**). However, the loss of basement membrane is not a necessary prerequisite for an invasive tumour. Sometimes there is an endogenous foreign body giant cell reaction to keratin (**14.11**) from ruptured pearls.

This tumour shows a moderately differentiated squamous cell carcinoma (**14.12**). It consists of small islands of squamous cells with a high mitotic index, nuclear hyperchromatism but no obvious keratinisation.

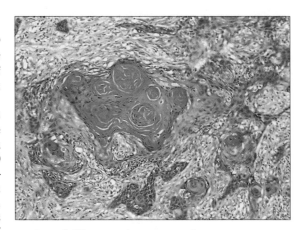

14.9 Well-differentiated squamous cell carcinoma.

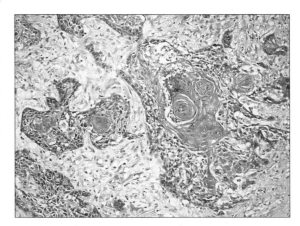

14.10 Well-differentiated squamous cell carcinoma.

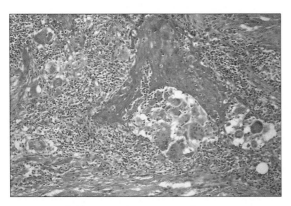

14.11 Well-differentiated squamous cell carcinoma showing giant cell reaction.

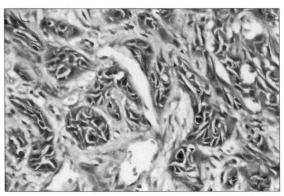

14.12 Moderatel differentiated squamous cell carcinoma.

14.13 illustrates a very poorly differentiated squamous cell carcinoma consisting of sheets of cells showing extreme pleomorphism, giant nuclei and multiple and bizarre mitoses. It is often difficult to distinguish these tumours from other malignancies, particularly poorly differentiated lymphomas or melanoma. Immunocytochemical markers such as keratins, common leukocyte antigen and melanoma-specific antibodies are then invaluable.

SPINDLE-CELL SQUAMOUS CARCINOMA

Rarely, oral squamous cell carcinomas consist predominantly, or entirely, of spindle-shaped cells. These often show pleomorphism and a high mitotic frequency (**14.14**). It may not be possible to diagnose poorly differentiated spindle-cell squamous carcinomas without immunocytochemical characterisation.

VERRUCOUS CARCINOMA

The verrucous carcinoma is a variant of oral squamous cell carcinoma. It tends to have a rather indolent course and presents as an exophytic mass typically with a warty or convoluted surface.

Microscopy shows gross acanthosis with the epithelium forming heaped-up folds but a low degree of epithelial atypia (**14.15**). Occasional cells show premature keratinisation although mitoses are rare. The advancing margin of the tumour tends to be at a single level, forming a so-called pushing margin rather than the typical finger-like invasion of a squamous cell carcinoma (**14.16**). Typically the epithelium is pulled up at the junction with the normal tissue, so the lesion is exophytic and the pushing margin of the tumour is often adjacent to the surrounding normal tissue. The underlying connective tissue may show dense chronic inflammation but this is variable. Eventually, after a protracted period, the tumour invades underlying tissues such as salivary glands and bone, but again usually as a unified pushing edge.

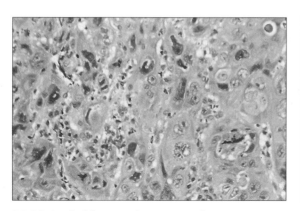

14.13 Poorly-differentiated squamous cell carcinoma.

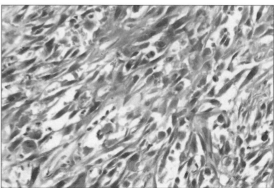

14.14 Spindle-cell squamous cell carcinoma.

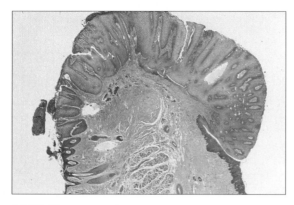

14.15 Verrucous carcinoma.

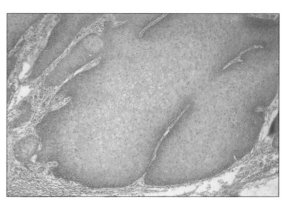

14.16 Verrucous carcinoma (higher power).

BASAL CELL CARCINOMA

Basal cell carcinomas originate from adnexal struc-tures of skin and are the most common malignant cutaneous tumours. They typically form a slow-growing, locally invasive nodule on the skin, partic-ularly in sun-exposed areas on the upper two-thirds of the face. If they ulcerate, they show a character-istically rolled, inverted margin.

The tumour is usually discrete and shows invasion of underlying tissues although usually to a fairly superficial level (it rarely invades the underlying muscle). The cells have variable morphology — they are usually small and basophilic, with a high nuclear-cytoplasmic ratio, and a high mitotic frequency. There may be palisading of the peripheral cells (**14.17**) and some tendency towards hair differentiation.

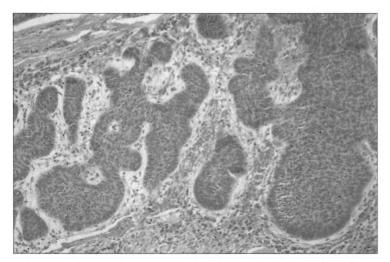

14.17 Basal cell carcinoma.

15.

SALIVARY DISEASES

ACUTE SIALADENITIS

Acute sialadenitis is much less common than formerly when it frequently followed abdominal surgery. It may be found in a previously normal gland as a result of ascending infection, often secondary to xerostomia or dehydration. Acute sialadenitis may also be found in patients who have organic disease of the salivary glands, particularly Sjögren's syndrome when there is also diminished salivary flow. Acute sialadenitis is typically seen in the parotid glands.

The diagnosis is usually made clinically and rarely involves microscopy. However, the example shown illustrates the extent of the potential destruction and emphasizes the need for rapid treatment. There are grossly dilated ducts filled with pus cells (neutrophils)

(15.1) and interstitial acute inflammation between the acinar cells, which are difficult to recognise. Focal aggregates of neutrophils are forming abscesses. This can only heal by fibrosis, resulting in loss of functional salivary tissue and distortion of the gland architecture which predisposes to further infection.

CHRONIC OBSTRUCTIVE SIALADENITIS

Chronic obstructive sialadenitis is considerably more common than acute sialadenitis. It is most often seen in the submandibular gland because this has a mucous secretion of moderately high viscosity while the duct is the longest of the salivary gland ducts. The main predisposing causes are obstruction, typically due to a stone, or fibrosis of the duct. Microscopically there is an extremely variable degree of inflammatory change, acinar destruction, and fibrosis — some glands which are very symptomatic appear almost normal when excised. Others show a considerable degree of damage. It is therefore very difficult to correlate the histopathology with the clinical symptoms.

This specimen shows a typical obstructed gland at a late stage, with dilatation of the larger ducts which may be filled with inspissated (dried-out) secretions (15.2, 15.3). Mucous or squamous metaplasia of the larger ducts is common, particularly if there is a stone in the duct. The smaller ducts are

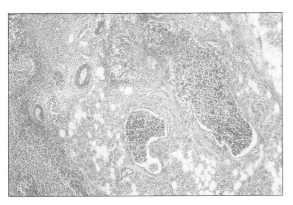

15.1 Acute sialadenitis.

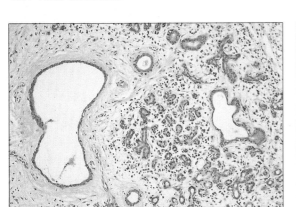

15.2 Chronic obstructive sialadenitis.

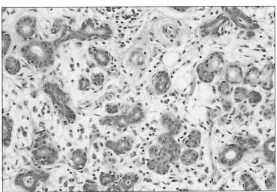

15.3 Chronic obstructive sialadenitis (higher power).

lined by cuboidal epithelium. There is extensive acinar atrophy and replacement by inflamed fibrous tissue. This is interstitial fibrosis with chronic interstitial inflammation. Around the smaller ducts, and some of the larger ducts, there may be periductal fibrosis.

Frequently, these glands appear to have more ducts than normal, probably due to de-differentiation of the acinar elements which then resemble ducts.

In the end-stages of the disease there is little remaining functional acinar tissue. These functionless glands are a liability to the patient, because they predispose to ascending infections. Eventually the gland is virtually replaced by fibrous tissue and becomes clinically hard and tumour-like (Küttner tumour).

SIALOSIS

Sialosis is an uncommon condition characterised by bilateral enlargement of the parotid glands. It is non-neoplastic and non-inflammatory and may be associated with a variety of factors including endocrine disorders, alcoholism, malnutrition (including bulimia) and drugs.

Microscopy shows hypertrophy of the serous cells which are usually granular, as shown, or occasionally vacuolated (**15.4**). There may be compression of the striated ducts and, in the later stages of the disease, extensive fatty replacement.

MUCOCELE

Probably 90–95% of mucoceles arise from ductal damage (extravasation mucoceles) and most are seen on the lower lip. **15.5** shows a typical early extravasation mucocele with mucus spilling out into the tissues from the damaged duct and evoking an acute inflammatory reaction with vascular hyperaemia, fibrin exudation and granulation tissue formation. Initially the lesion is diffuse and may be dismissed microscopically as an acute inflammatory lesion or merely granulation tissue. However, under higher power there are foamy macrophages which are macrophages that have ingested mucus (muciphages) (**15.6**).

At a later stage, there is much less inflammation in the surrounding tissues because the mucocele is

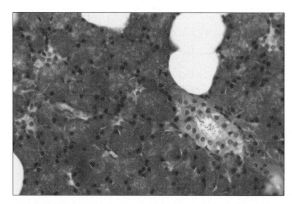

15.4 Sialosis.

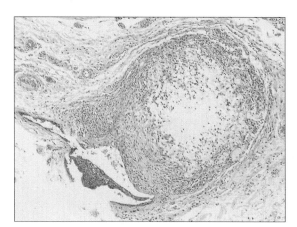

15.5 Extravasation mucocele.

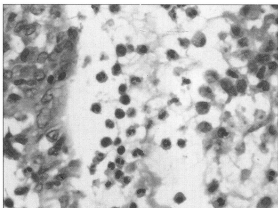

15.6 Extravasation mucocele (higher power).

walled off by fibrous tissue (**15.7**). The cyst is lined by mucus-containing macrophages which in some cases resemble epithelial cells. These lesions may thus be easily confused with retention mucoceles (**15.8**). However, staining for reticulin shows that there is no basement membrane zone. When reporting these lesions, the presence or absence of the adjacent minor gland should be recorded because if the surgeon removes the mucocele but leaves the damaged gland there may be recurrence. Similarly, recurrence may also follow damage to an adjacent gland during excision.

Some mucoceles are so superficial that they produce a subepithelial or intraepithelial blister (**15.9**). These often present clinically as multiple or recurrent intraoral small tense blisters which rupture to leave superficial ulcers that then rapidly heal. The importance of superficial mucoceles is that they can be mistaken microscopically for vesiculo-bullous lesions such as mucous membrane pemphigoid and pemphigus vulgaris.

Retention mucoceles are most common in the floor of the mouth, in relation to the sublingual gland (ranula). They are typically non-inflamed and lined by attenuated epithelium which may be columnar or occasionally stratified (**15.10**). It is important for the pathologist to examine such lesions carefully, because salivary gland tumours, both benign and malignant, can present with a significant cystic component. Because the tumour may only be a small area of mural thickening in a cyst it is easy to miss. Therefore, it is essential to examine the whole specimen and not just assume that the lesion is a cyst.

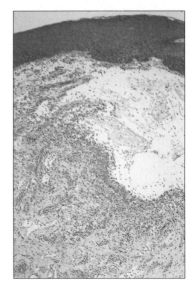

15.7 Extravasation mucocele.

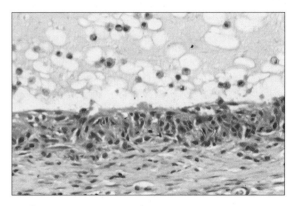

15.8 Extravasation mucocele.

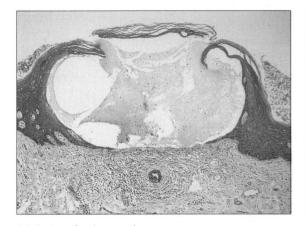

15.9 Superficial mucocele.

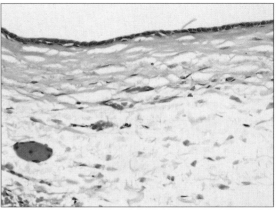

15.10 Retention mucocele.

SJÖGREN'S SYNDROME

Sjögren's syndrome is an autoimmune inflammatory exocrinopathy with multisystem manifestations, particularly xerostomia and sometimes salivary gland swelling.

Initially, focal periductal lymphocytic sialadenitis is seen, typically with some proliferation of the ducts as shown in a submandibular gland from Sjögren's syndrome (**15.11**). The lymphocytes spread centrifugally from the duct into the surrounding acinar tissue which just seems to dissolve away without showing clear signs of cell death. At the same time, the ducts start to proliferate to form so-called epimyoepithelial islands.

The lymphocytic infiltrate then spreads through the lobule of the gland and completely replaces the acinar tissue (**5.12**). The ducts proliferate and become solid, so that in the plane of section they appear as islands which, as they are said to contain myoepithelial cells, are called epimyoepithelial islands (**15.13**). This type of appearance is seen in Sjögren's syndrome and in so-called lymphoepithelial lesions or myoepithelial sialadenitis (MESA). The islands often contain variable amounts of pink, hyalinised material which is basement membrane material including laminin and type IV collagen which

has been elaborated by the proliferating cells. The islands are frequently infiltrated by lymphocytes.

The fact that the lymphocytic infiltrate is limited by the fibrous septa of the gland is important to note when examining these lesions because during progression to lymphoma (a complication of Sjögren's syndrome), one of the first events is obliteration of the fibrous septa by the infiltrate.

Typically, the major glands show virtual destruction of all the acinar tissue. One of the potential problems in interpreting the findings in major glands is the presence of superimposed ascending bacterial infection, particularly in the later stages, because the gland secretion has been compromised by extensive acinar loss. This can lead to chronic non-specific sialadenitis.

Changes in the minor (labial) salivary glands mirror those in the major salivary glands and they are frequently biopsied as part of the investigation. **15.14** shows a typical labial salivary gland biopsy specimen from a patient with Sjögren's syndrome. There is focal periductal inflammatory infiltration which is predominantly lymphocytic and some interstitial inflammation which is again largely lymphocytic with occasional plasma cells. The ducts are normal (it is uncommon to see any ductal proliferation in minor glands).

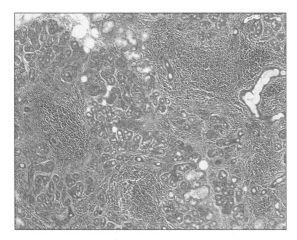

15.11 Sjögren's syndrome.

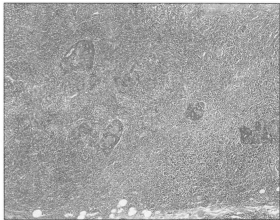

15.12 Sjögren's syndrome.

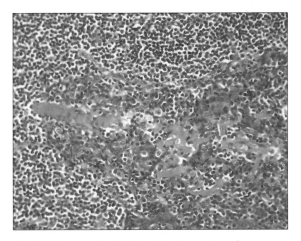

15.13 Epimyoepithelial islands in Sjögren's syndrome.

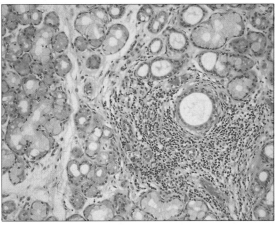

15.14 Labial salivary gland biopsy in Sjögren's syndrome.

NECROTISING SIALOMETAPLASIA

Necrotising sialometaplasia is typically seen in the palate, although it can also be found in other minor and occasionally major salivary glands. It presents as a nondescript lump or ulcer which, if left alone, usually heals spontaneously within one to three months, depending on its size. The main problem with this lesion is that clinically and histologically it can simulate malignancy and lead to an erroneous diagnosis of cancer — usually squamous cell carcinoma or mucoepidermoid carcinoma.

The cause of the condition is unknown, but there may be a history of trauma or heavy smoking. It is possibly related to ischaemia. The primary event seems to be damage to the minor glands which undergo necrosis (infarction) (**15.15, 15.16**). At the periphery of the necrotic area there is inflammation while the adjacent salivary ducts undergo regenerative hyperplasia and become solid, and show squamous metaplasia.

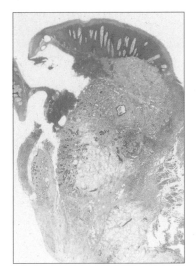

15.15 Necrotising sialometaplasia.

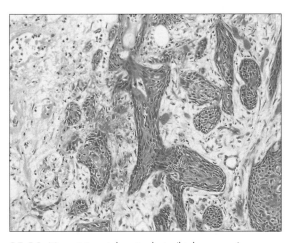

15.16 Necrotising sialometaplasia (higher power).

PLEOMORPHIC SALIVARY ADENOMA

The pleomorphic salivary adenoma (PSA) is the most common salivary neoplasm and is seen mainly in the parotid gland. PSAs are benign tumours which are characterised microscopically by an extreme degree of architectural pleomorphism. They do not, however, have cellular pleomorphism (in which case they would be characterised as malignant) but show a very wide variety of cellular differentiation and architectural configurations.

The two main elements of the PSA are epithelial and stromal. The epithelial elements can form sheets, duct-like structures which may be part of a sheet, or separate duct-like structures sometimes with an architecture resembling intercalated ducts with inner duct-lining cells and outer clear myoepithelial cells (**15.17**). It is not uncommon for the epithelial cells to show squamous metaplasia, with or without keratin pearl formation (**15.18**). In contrast, mucoepidermoid carcinomas contain keratin pearls only in exceptional circumstances.

The duct-like structures in PSA often contain eosinophilic material which sometimes forms discrete structures similar to the corpora amylacea of the prostate gland. The PSA may show plasmacytoid (hyaline) cells which are thought to be myoepithelial (**15.19**).

The connective tissue component of PSAs is either mucoid (sometimes called myxoid) and rich in glycosaminoglycans with few associated cells, or chondroid with cartilaginous differentiation (**15.20**). This is true cartilage which will stain with S100 or keratan sulphate proteoglycan. Osseous metaplasia may also be seen. Elastic-tissue formation is often found in the stroma and stains intensely pink and homogeneously with haematoxylin and eosin stain. As these tumours mature, the epithelial component becomes less conspicuous as the fibrosis increases.

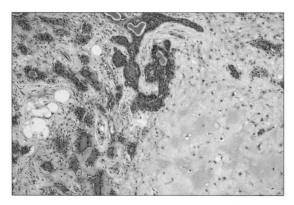

15.17 Pleomorphic adenoma.

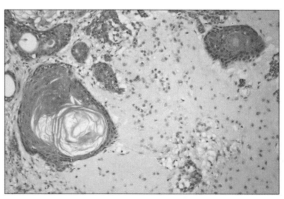

15.18 Pleomorphic adenoma (squamous metaplasia).

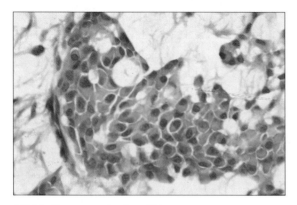

15.19 Plasmacytoid cells in PSA.

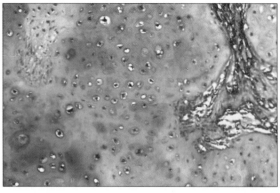

15.20 Pleomorphic adenoma showing cartilaginous differentiation.

It is particularly important to scrutinise closely these scarred tumours because malignant change can often arise within the scarred tissue.

Occasionally there is increased mitotic activity and/or evidence of pleomorphism within the substance of the tumour which then becomes classified as a non-invasive carcinoma (which is almost a contradiction in terms) (**15.21**). This may be a precursor stage of carcinoma in pleomorphic adenoma and is probably better termed 'dysplastic pleomorphic adenoma'. Usually the whole tumour has been removed and there is no evidence that the prognosis is changed.

Pleomorphic adenomas, particularly in the parotid gland, tend to recur and may become malignant with time. Recurrence is, however, extremely variable and ranges between 3 and 10% over 10–20 years (the longer the follow up, the higher the recurrence rate). The rate of malignant transformation is also variable and lies between 5 and 10% (again the risk increases with duration).

The tendency for pleomorphic adenomas to recur is mainly related to the morphology of the tumour. This is represented diagramatically in **15.22**. There is often a compressed fibrous tissue capsule although this is highly variable in thickness and may be absent in places. In addition, the tumour tends to invade the capsule (**15.23**) and may bulge through it while remaining attached to the main tumour mass by a small isthmus (although this may not be apparent in the plane of section) (**15.24**). It is easy to leave these bulging pieces of tumour *in situ* during attempts at local excision. The tumour may show a plane of cleavage between the capsule and the tumour which results in dissociation from the capsule during the

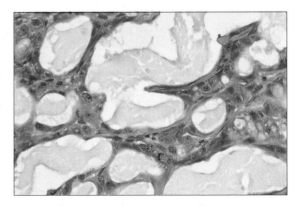

15.21 Pleomorphic adenoma showing dysplasia.

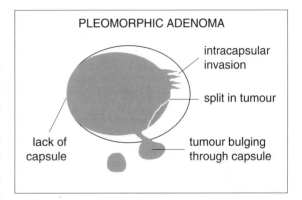

15.22 Pleomorphic adenoma.

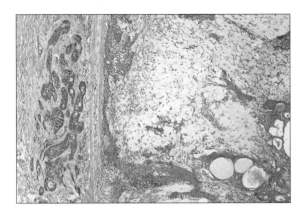

15.23 Pleomorphic adenoma.

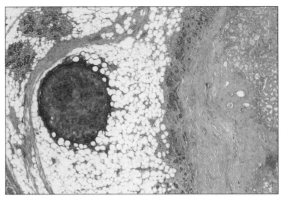

15.24 Pleomorphic adenoma.

operative procedure (at one time these tumours were shelled out). However, remaining fragments of capsule may have adherent tumour (because the plane of cleavage is actually within the tumour) and recurrence may follow. The other reason that PSAs tend to recur is that some of the cells, particularly in the myxoid and cartilaginous elements, probably have fairly low nutritional requirements (most other tumour cells left *in situ* will die because they need a richer blood supply). Tumours which are predominantly myxoid are said to have a high rate of recurrence, probably because they easily rupture and spill into the wound during surgery. If recurrence ensues, multiple tumours tend to develop which may be impossible to eradicate — patients can die from such uncontrolled benign tumours (**15.25**). The histology of the recurrent tumour often bears little relationship to that of the original tumour. The recurrent lesion could be solid and the original tumour myxoid, or vice versa.

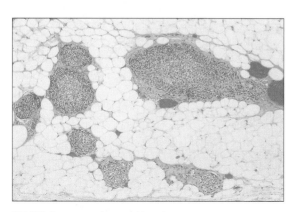

15.25 Recurrent pleomorphic adenoma.

WARTHIN'S TUMOUR (ADENO-LYMPHOMA OR PAPILLARY CYS-TADENOMA LYMPHOMATOSUM)

Warthin's tumour is a benign neoplasm which develops almost exclusively in the parotid gland. It is thought that these tumours arise from ectopic salivary gland tissue within intra- or paraparotid lymph nodes. It is common to find salivary gland inclusions in lymph nodes related to the parotid gland and transitions between these inclusions and classical Warthin's tumours are sometimes seen. An interesting feature of Warthin's tumours is the change in the male to female incidence ratio. In the first large survey in the 1950s, there was a male to female ratio of about 10:1 which is still quoted in many text books. However, all the recent large surveys show a more or less equal sex ratio.

Warthin's tumours have a very characteristic histological appearance resulting from two main components, epithelial and lymphoid (**15.26**). The epithelium typically forms cysts, often with papillary processes extending into them. The cysts usually contain a glairy, gelatinous fluid. The epithelium lining the cysts is oncocytic — the cells are pink and granular on haematoxylin and eosin staining (**15.27**). The cysts have a luminal layer of tall columnar cells with regular palisaded nuclei, and a basal layer of cells which is much less regular (**15.28**). It is common to see so-called apocrine blebs on the luminal aspect but cilia are much less frequent. The oncocytic cells comprise two cell types (as do all oncocytic tumours): light cells, which have rather vesicular nuclei and moderately oncocytic, granular cytoplasm, and the much less numerous dark cells, which have a deeply basophilic shrunken nucleus and much denser cytoplasm. These dark cells are probably effete forms of

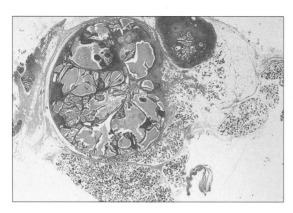

15.26 Warthin's tumour.

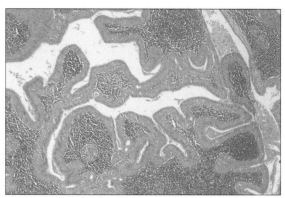

15.27 Warthin's tumour.

the light cells and are sometimes seen extruding into the cyst cavity. These tumours often have focal areas of mucous metaplasia and, less frequently, squamous metaplasia. This can occasionally lead to a mistaken diagnosis of mucoepidermoid carcinoma. This can happen particularly if the gland becomes inflamed, or infarcts and becomes fibrotic.

The lymphoid component of Warthin's tumour is normal lymphoid tissue showing germinal centres and frequently a typical lymph-node structure, such as a capsule around the outside of the tumour and a subcapsular sinus.

15.29 shows a normal lymph node which had a subcapsular sinus and typical lymphoid structure. There are oncocytic salivary gland inclusions and an early Warthin's tumour. These findings are used to support the previously mentioned hypothesis that Warthin's tumours arise from ectopic salivary tissue within intra- or paraparotid lymph nodes. However, Warthin's tumours sometimes lack typical lymph-node structure or are in direct continuity with the surrounding gland. In other cases there is so much lymphoid tissue that the Warthin's tumour could not have arisen from a normal lymph node, because the volume is too great. A combination of factors may be involved — Warthin's tumours may arise from salivary inclusions within lymph nodes and then cause reactive hyperplasia.

OTHER ADENOMAS

There is a variety of benign salivary gland neoplasms which were once grouped under the designation 'monomorphic adenomas'. The tendency is now to give each type of tumour a specific name. The most important tumours are basal cell adenomas and canalicular adenomas. Both tumours can affect either major or minor glands, although the canalicular adenoma is seen almost exclusively in the latter. Upper-lip salivary gland tumours are 10-fold more common than tumours in the lower lip, for reasons which are unknown. The most common tumour in the upper lip is the canalicular adenoma.

The **canalicular adenoma** usually presents as a swelling which is often cystic and may be mistaken for a mucocele. The diagnostic difficulty is some-times compounded because the lesion may be nearly all cyst with the tumour forming only a small mural thickening. The tumour consists of interlacing cords of columnar epithelium, with areas of stromal degen-eration showing surviving blood vessels within the stroma (**15.30**). There is no evidence of mitotic activity in these tumours. Canalicular adenomas are usually well encapsulated and tend not to recur.

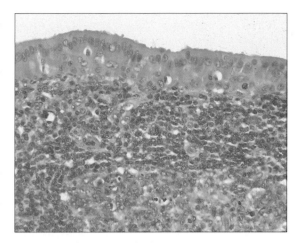

15.28 Warthin's tumour (higher power).

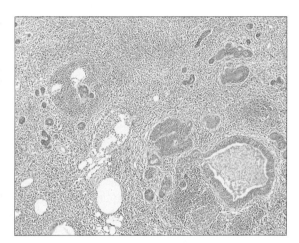

15.29 Warthin's tumour developing from rests within a lymph node.

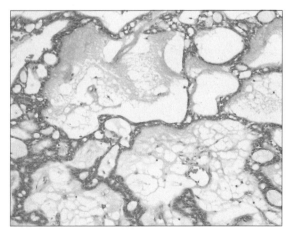

15.30 Canalicular adenoma.

Basal cell adenomas show a variety of appearances but the most common consists of dark-staining cells in a tubulo-trabecular configuration in a fibrous or fibroblastic stroma (**15.31**). These tumours are predominantly seen in the parotid gland.

The **oncocytoma** is a rare tumour which again arises in the parotid gland of elderly patients. Microscopy shows sheets or groups of granular, eosinophilic cells sometimes showing duct-like spaces (**15.32**). Typically there are variable numbers of cells with dark, pyknotic nuclei and condensed cytoplasm — so-called dark cells. Many benign and malignant salivary gland tumours can either show focal areas of oncocytosis or be entirely oncocytic. These changes are more common than true oncocytoma.

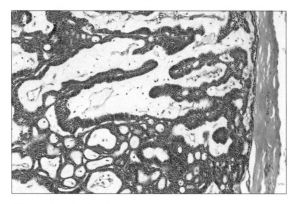

15.31 Basal cell adenoma.

MUCOEPIDERMOID CARCINOMA (MUCOEPIDERMOID TUMOUR)

Some large surveys show the mucoepidermoid carcinoma to be the most frequent intraoral malignant salivary gland neoplasm although other studies imply that it is uncommon. There seems to be a relatively higher frequency in the USA than in Europe. Although mucoepidermoid carcinomas often clinically appear circumscribed, histologically this is rarely the case. They have no capsule and usually possess a very irregular margin.

Mucoepidermoid carcinomas consist predominantly of two cell types in varying proportions and configurations: epidermoid (or squamous cells) and mucous cells. There is also another cell, an intermediate cell, which is thought to be a precursor of both the mucous and epidermoid types, but intermediate cells are often relatively inconspicuous.

The most common appearance is of islands and sheets of epithelial cells with variable degrees of cyst formation (**15.33, 15.34**). Frequently, the cysts are

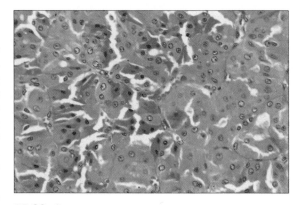

15.32 Oncocytoma.

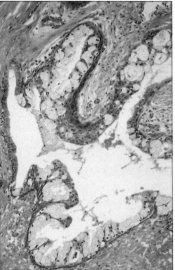

15.34 Mucoepidermoid carcinoma (higher power).

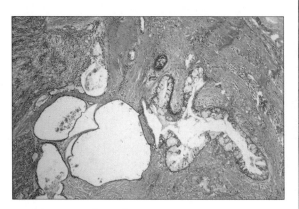

15.33 Mucoepidermoid carcinoma.

lined with epidermoid cells. Intermingled with epidermoid cells are mucous cells (**15.35**), some of which contain obvious mucous droplets while others are clear with rigid cell boundaries and a peripheral nucleus (clear cell variant) (**15.36**).

The stroma is usually fibrous, and inflammatory changes are common because mucus tends to spill into the adjacent tissues. Sometimes cholesterol clefts are seen in addition to foreign body giant cell reactions to the tumour.

Mucoepidermoid carcinomas can be graded into well-differentiated (low-grade) and poorly differentiated (high-grade) tumours. The low-grade tumours tend to be predominantly mucous and cystic, whereas the high-grade lesions tend to be predominantly epidermoid and solid. Tumours which are predominantly squamous often resemble squamous cell carcinomas but keratin pearl formation is virtually never seen and special stains may be necessary to highlight mucous cells. These tumours are aggressive and tend to recur or metastasise. The main problem in predicting behaviour is with the well-differentiated tumours; the majority of 'low-grade' tumours behave like pleomorphic adenomas with local invasion and local recurrence, but some unpredictably metastasise.

ACINIC CELL CARCINOMA (ACINIC CELL TUMOUR)

The acinic cell carcinoma is a tumour of intermediate behaviour. It consists of cells that closely resemble normal salivary acinar cells. In well-differentiated tumours the cells are basophilic and granular and possess cytoplasmic granules which resemble and stain in exactly the same way as the zymogen granules of normal serous cells.

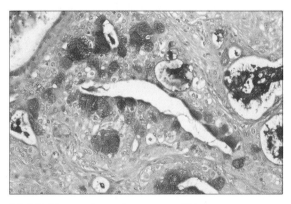

15.35 Mucoepidermoid carcinoma. PAS stain.

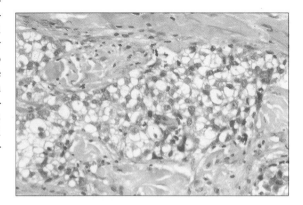

15.36 Mucoepidermoid carcinoma — clear cell variant.

These tumours have a variety of different configurations and degrees of differentiation. The most common type, shown here, consists of cells which resemble normal acinar cells arranged in sheets. There are spaces within the sheets of cells which are not duct-like but contain secreted material (**15.37, 15.38**).

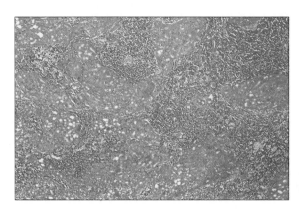

15.37 Acinic cell carcinoma.

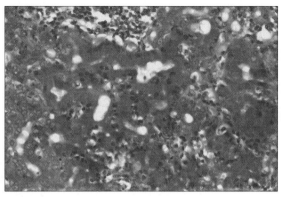

15.38 Acinic cell carcinoma (higher power).

This produces a microcystic pattern within the tumour. Sometimes the microcysts become more conspicuous and start to fuse and form larger cysts (when the tumour may resemble a follicular thyroid carcinoma). Psammoma bodies, which are concentrically laminated calcifications, are not infrequently found. They can sometimes be detected on fine needle aspiration cytology and may help confirm the diagnosis. Clear cell change is another feature of acinic cell carcinomas and these lesions come into the differential diagnosis of clear cell tumours of salivary glands. Another feature is that approximately 3% of tumours are bilateral. Some acinic cell carcinomas have a florid lymphocytic infiltrate so that they appear as if they have metastasised to a lymph node.

The majority of acinic cell carcinomas show limited local invasion and are relatively easily excised. The morphology of these tumours, however, does not correlate well with their behaviour — even well-differentiated tumours can unpredictably metastasise.

ADENOID CYSTIC CARCINOMA

Adenoid cystic carcinomas are the most common malignant intraoral salivary gland tumours in the UK. They have a tendency to undergo perineural spread and often advance far beyond the clinical estimation of the margins of the tumour. They grow very slowly but occasionally, because of perineural spread, it is impossible to eradicate the tumour surgically. Adenoid cystic carcinomas are radiosensitive although radiation merely slows their progress. After five years most patients with adenoid cystic carcinoma are alive and well, but by 15–20 years most have died as a result of, or with, the tumour.

Adenoid cystic carcinomas can show a variety of different growth patterns including cribriform, tubular and solid. **15.39** shows the classical so-called 'Swiss-cheese' or cylindromatous pattern. There are islands of small, angular cells which have a dark nucleus and clear cytoplasm. Typically, duct-lining cells are also seen within these islands. It is very uncommon to see any mitoses in these tumours. The spaces or cylinders usually contain either ground substance or basement membrane material and elastic tissue which has been elaborated by the tumour.

The other feature is the tendency of the tumours to undergo perineural and intraneural spread (**15.40**). Typically, these tumours spread in this way by nerves or, in the late stage of the disease, they may show

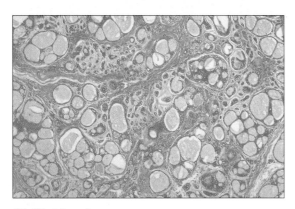

15.39 Adenoid cystic carcinoma.

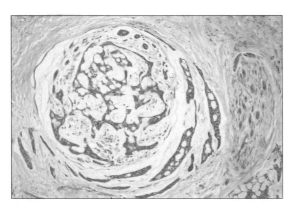

15.40 Adenoid cystic carcinoma showing neural invasion.

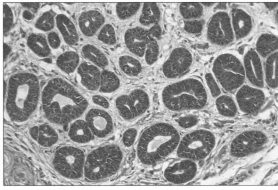

15.41 Adenoid cystic carcinoma — tubular variant.

distant spread to the bones and lungs. There may also be lymph-node involvement but this is not usually via lymphatic embolisation or permeation but rather by contiguous expansion of the tumour into an adjacent lymph node.

Tubular variants consist typically of double-layered duct-like structures. Sometimes cells in the outer layer have a clear cytoplasm and appear to be myoepithelial (**15.41**). The tubular type is the most clearly differentiated variant and has the most favourable prognosis, the cylindromatous variant has an intermediate prognosis.

ADENOID CYSTIC CARCINOMA (SOLID VARIANT)

On initial examination, the solid variant of adenoid cystic carcinoma seems to bear little resemblance to classical adenoid cystic carcinoma. There are solid islands of tumour which often undergo central (comedo) necrosis (**15.42**). The cells are small, dark and rather angular and may show mitoses. Ductal differentiation tends to be seen within these islands so that small lumina appear (**15.43**). These are the same type of duct-like structures described within cylindromatous areas, lined by columnar cells. It is important to distinguish the solid variant of adenoid cystic carcinoma from a range of other baseloid tumours. The solid type of adenoid cystic carcinoma is the most aggressive variant.

One of the problems encountered when trying to make a prognostic judgement based on histology, is that the prognosis is also dependent on a multitude of other factors which include the size of the tumour, its site, growth rate, nerve involvement, metastases, treatment and age of the patient. However, as a general rule, adenoid cystic carcinomas which are predominantly solid (or even those which have any significant amount of solid tissue) tend to have a much worse prognosis than the tubular or cylindromatous types.

ADENOCARCINOMA (NOT OTHERWISE SPECIFIED)

Adenocarcinomas occasionally show ductal differentiation but no other specific features (**15.44**).

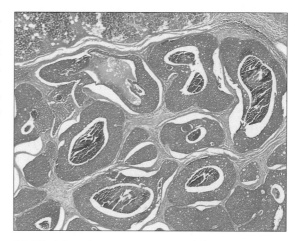

15.42 Adenoid cystic carcinoma — solid variant.

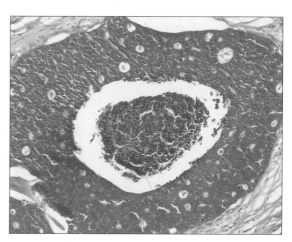

15.43 Adenoid cystic carcinoma — solid variant (higher power).

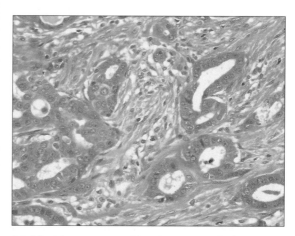

15.44 Adenocarcinoma (not otherwise specified).

POLYMORPHOUS LOW-GRADE ADENOCARCINOMA (TERMINAL DUCT CARCINOMA)

This is a relatively uncommon carcinoma which arises almost exclusively in minor glands, particularly of the palate. It is characterised by its morphological diversity and cytological uniformity. The cells appear bland, i.e. show little atypia and few mitoses. On the other hand, there is a wide variety of architectural configurations including lobular, cribriform, tubular and papillary areas (**15.45–15.47**). Some tumours show striking neurotropism and cells which are concentrically laminated around nerves produce a targetoid appearance (**15.48**). The stroma shows areas of mucinosis and hyalinisation (**15.47**). Despite the resemblance of some tumours to adenoid cystic carcinoma, particularly the perineural invasion, these tumours are low-grade. They tend to show limited local spread and often respond to conservative local excision. Polymorphous low-grade adenocarcinomas rarely metastasise therefore giving a better prognosis than suggested by their histological appearance.

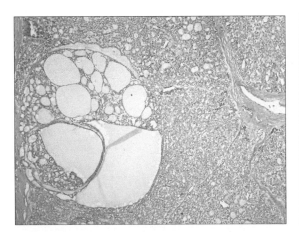

15.45 Polymorphous low-grade adenocarcinoma.

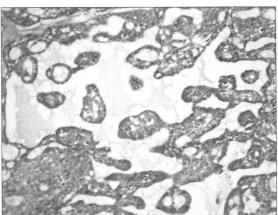

15.46 Polymorphous low-grade adenocarcinoma.

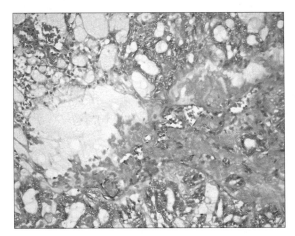

15.47 Polymorphous low-grade adenocarcinoma.

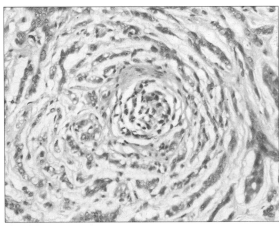

15.48 Polymorphous low-grade adenocarcinoma.

EPITHELIAL-MYOEPITHELIAL CARCINOMA (INTERCALATED DUCT CARCINOMA)

This is an uncommon but characteristic tumour which is found predominantly in the parotid and sub-mandibular glands. In the past it was classified as an adenoma (clear cell adenoma or glycogen-rich adenoma). It is now recognised, however, that despite the tumour's often bland histology, recurrence and metastasis are not uncommon.

Epithelial–myoepithelial carcinomas consist of two cell types in varying proportions and configurations which may form duct-like structures. They possess inner, small, dark-staining cells and an outer layer of clear cells (**15.49**). The outer cells often stain for glycogen with PAS (**15.50**) and are also positive with S100 (**15.51**), actin and myosin stains, confirming their myoepithelial origin. Sometimes the clear cells predominate, and form sheets of cells with only sparse ductal structures. Mitoses are infrequent but there may be evidence of neural or vascular invasion. Approximately one-third of these tumours recur locally or metastasise.

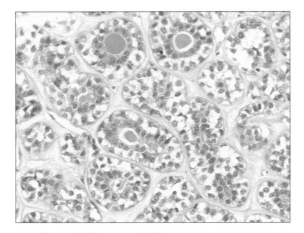

15.49 Epithelial–myoepithelial carcinoma.

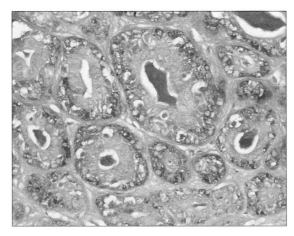

15.50 Epithelial-myoepithelial carcinoma. PAS stain.

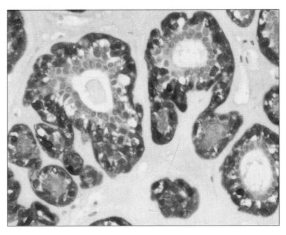

15.51 Epithelial-myoepithelial carcinoma. S100 stain.

CARCINOMA IN PLEOMORPHIC ADENOMA

Between 5 and 10% of pleomorphic adenomas eventually become malignant. Some tumours show an area of typical pleomorphic adenoma with carcinomatous elements in direct juxtaposition. However, in many cases the tumour arises in an area of lesion scarring, so that the original pleomorphic adenoma has disappeared. Alternatively, the carcinomatous elements overgrow the original tumour. **15.52** shows a pleomorphic adenoma with juxtaposed malignant elements. There is a typical pleomorphic salivary adenoma with chondromyxoid stroma and double-layered duct-like structures on the left. The cells are about three times larger in the adjacent area of adenocarcinoma (right), and there are frequent mitoses.

Some carcinomas in pleomorphic adenomas show several different types of differentiation such as an adenocarcinoma and a squamous cell carcinoma — either in separate areas of the tumour or intermingled. This combination of several different tumour types within a single mass is very typical of this condition.

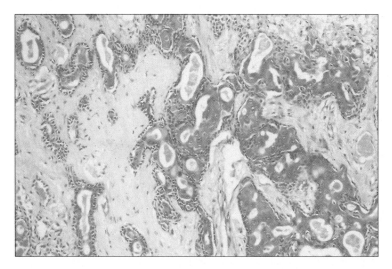

15.52 Carcinoma in pleomorphic adenoma.

16.

LYMPHORETICULAR DISEASES

CAT SCRATCH DISEASE

Cat scratch disease results from an infection by a pleomorphic bacillus (*Afipia felis*), usually secondary to a scratch from a cat. It produces tender cervical lymphadenopathy and fever (the latter particularly in children).

The lymph-node biopsy appearance shown in **16.1** is characteristic of the early stages, but later may resemble tuberculosis. There are discrete, epithelioid granulomas of the so-called palisading type (when the macrophages tend to line up like spokes of a wheel from the centre of the granuloma) (**16.1**), and multinucleated giant cells. However, one of the most characteristic features of the early stages is suppuration at the centre of the granuloma, which is filled with polymorphs.

At a later stage, the suppuration is less conspicuous and discrete epithelioid granulomas with central areas that resemble tuberculous caseation make microscopical distinction between the conditions quite difficult (**16.2**). Eventually the suppuration resolves and the lesion heals spontaneously by fibrosis.

LYMPHOMAS

In the head and neck region, lymphomas mainly affect the cervical lymph nodes but can involve the salivary glands or be seen intraorally, typically in the fauces or palate. Lymphomas are a complex and contentious area of pathology, with classifications that have been changing radically over the last two decades. Some of these classifications are based on the morphological features of the tumour while others are based on the immuno-cytochemical features. It is inappropriate to discuss this specialist area of pathology in detail here.

From a practical point-of-view, lymphomas are divided into two main groups — Hodgkin's disease and non-Hodgkin's lymphoma. The cell of origin in Hodgkin's disease is uncertain, but is likely to be an undifferentiated cell of lymphocytic type rather than of macrophage lineage. Non-Hodgkin's lymphomas arise mainly from B lymphocytes although it is being increasing recognised that many intraoral lymphomas are of T-cell origin.

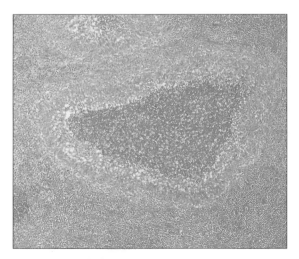

16.1 Cat scratch disease.

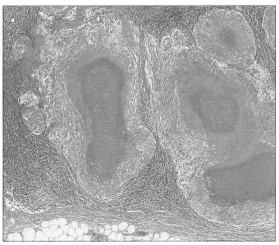

16.2 Cat scratch disease.

NON-HODGKIN'S LYMPHOMA

The classification of non-Hodgkin's lymphoma is complex, but essentially the prognosis depends on the morphology of the cells and their configuration, particularly whether they form follicles. Non-Hodgkin's lymphomas can therefore be divided into two main groups — diffuse and follicular. Within each of those groups, lymphomas are classified according to whether the cells are poorly or well differentiated. They can be characterised more precisely by immuno-cytochemical techniques.

16.3 shows a lymphoma consisting of a diffuse sheet of small uniform lymphocytes, with occasional mitoses. The specimen is well differentiated, with pachychromatic nuclei and nuclear chromatin, and no significant cytoplasmic component which would suggest plasmacytoid differentiation. Staining for kappa and lambda immunoglobulin light chains (light chain restriction) may help differentiate macro-

phages from centroblasts. This specimen shows virtually all the cells to be positive for kappa chains, indicating monoclonality (**16.4**). In extra-nodal lymphomas of the head and neck, there is usually so much inflammatory reaction that the lesion is polyclonal; in these circumstances, staining for kappa or lambda chains is not really helpful. In lymph nodes, however, monoclonality is supportive of the diagnosis of lymphoma as opposed to reactive hyperplasia.

16.5 shows a follicular lymphoma in a lymph node. The macrophages with tingible bodies, which are present within normal germinal centres, are not apparent and there is no rim of compressed lymphocytes around each of the nodules. Indeed, some nodules are tending to fuse with each other. A reticulin stain outlines the fibrous tissue around the follicles or nodules and usually shows them quite clearly, even when they are less conspicuous than shown here (**16.6**). A less well-differentiated follicular lymphoma consisting of a mixture of centroblasts

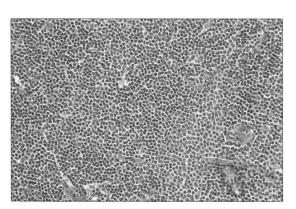

16.3 Lymphocytic lymphoma — well differentiated and diffuse.

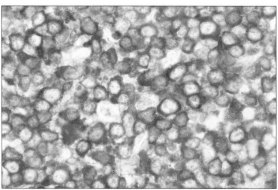

16.4 Monoclonal staining for Kappa light chain. Immunoperoxidase stain.

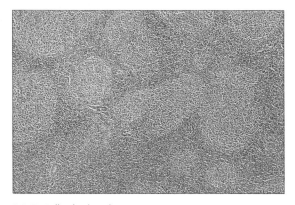

16.5 Follicular lymphoma.

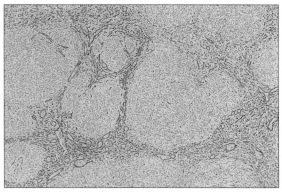

16.6 Follicular lymphoma. Reticulin stain.

and centrocytes is shown in **16.7**. Sometimes there is no need to treat these lymphomas as they can remain static for years before entering a phase when they become diffuse and show accelerated growth. Alternatively, they may progress to a leukaemic phase with chronic lymphatic leukaemia. Elderly patients with this type of lymphoma may well die from intercurrent disease rather than the lymphoma.

Both follicular and diffuse non-Hodgkin's lymphomas can arise intraorally, most commonly at the junction between the hard and soft palate. Lymphoid infiltrates in extra-nodal sites can be difficult to interpret because the normal lymph-node structure is unavailable for comparison. In **16.8**, the lymphoid infiltrate is obviously more than reactive because it is infiltrating and destroying both muscle and nerve.

BURKITT'S LYMPHOMA

This lymphoma is endemic in parts of East Africa and probably results from the Epstein–Barr virus. It is multifocal and multicentric, predominantly affecting children. The jaws are the site of presentation in about half of the cases when they develop rapidly progressive osteolytic lesions. Burkitt's lymphoma typically shows a good response to chemotherapy.

Microscopy shows sheets of undifferentiated, small cells derived from B lymphocytes together with scattered histiocytes with pale vacuolated cytoplasm which gives the tumour its characteristic 'starry sky' pattern (**16.9**).

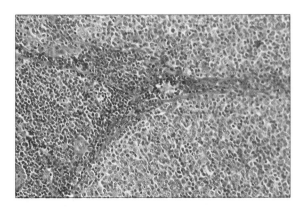

16.7 Follicular lymphoma (higher power).

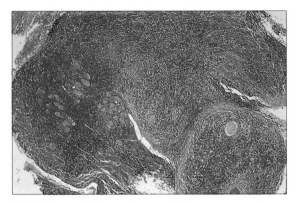

16.8 Extra-nodal diffuse lymphocytic lymphoma.

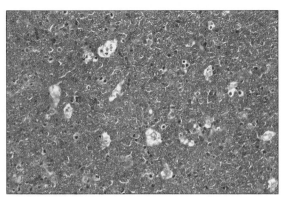

16.9 Burkitt's lymphoma.

HODGKIN'S DISEASE

The classification of Hodgkin's disease has, until fairly recently, been far more straightforward than that of non-Hodgkin's lymphoma.

There are four main types of Hodgkin's disease. The commonest is the lymphocyte-predominant type when most of the involved tissue comprises small lymphocytes with few of the pathognomonic cells of Hodgkin's disease (Reed–Sternberg cells or Sternberg-Reed cells) (**16.10**). These are large cells, typically with mirror-image double nuclei, each with a prominent nuclear membrane and a prominent nucleolus. The presence of few Reed–Sternberg cells is typical of lymphocyte-predominant Hodgkin's disease.

In classical Hodgkin's disease (mixed-cellularity Hodgkin's disease) there is a much more pleomorphic cellular infiltrate, with moderate numbers of Reed-Sternberg cells and often many eosinophils (**16.11**).

There can also be large multinucleated cells, variants of Reed-Sternberg cells, which are called megakaryocytoid giant cells. These cells are said to look like coins on a plate because of their overlapping nuclei (**16.12**). Sometimes there is a tendency to form epithelioid granulomas, which may occasionally be quite striking, and this can mask the underlying disease process.

In nodular sclerosing Hodgkin's disease, the node tends to be split by fibrous septa into irregular nodules. The Reed-Sternberg cells tend to lie in spaces and become known as lacunar cells (**16.13**). Athough these are not pathognomonic of nodular sclerosing Hodgkin's disease, they are most consistently seen in this variant.

At the most malignant end of the spectrum is lymphocyte-depleted Hodgkin's disease, which usually involves very extensive fibrosis, pleomorphism, frequent mitoses and few lymphocytes (**16.14**).

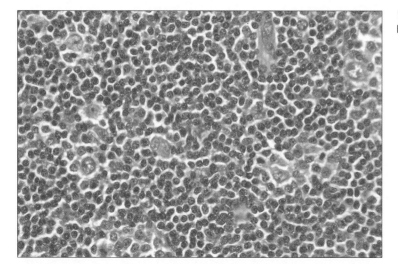

16.10 Lymphocyte predominant Hodgkin's disease.

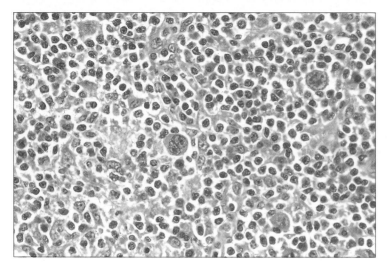

16.11 Mixed cellularity Hodgkin's disease.

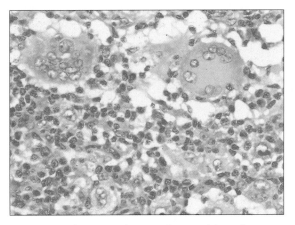

16.12 Megakaryocytoid giant cells in Hodgkin's disease.

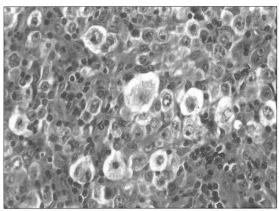

16.13 Nodular sclerosing Hodgkin's disease.

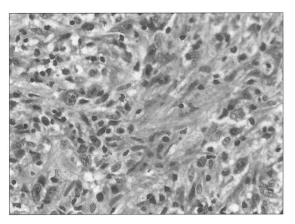

16.14 Lymphocyte-depleted Hodgkin's disease.

PLASMACYTOMA AND MYELOMA

Plasmacytomas are solitary lesions consisting of malignant plasma cells seen mainly in soft tissues and occasionally in bone. They may be isolated, but often patients who have solitary plasmacytomas develop multiple myeloma after many years. The histology of plasmacytoma is identical to multiple myeloma. There is a destructive lesion consisting of plasma cells of varying degrees of differentiation. These plasma cells are usually easily recognisable, even though they are abnormal and show variation in shape and size (**16.15**). In poorly differentiated tumours some of the cells have multiple nuclei, others are binucleated and there are many mitoses (**16.16**).

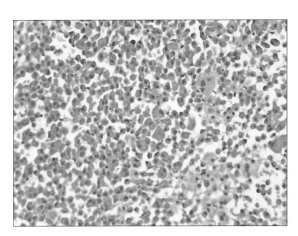

16.15 Well-differentiated plasmacytoma.

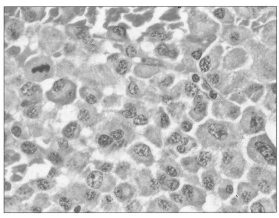

16.16 Poorly differentiated plasmacytoma (high power).

AMYLOIDOSIS

Amyloid is a fibrillar, insoluble protein which can be deposited in tissues in a variety of pathological conditions. There are two main types: primary amyloidosis, which is related to multiple myeloma or an abnormal but benign clone of plasma cells; and secondary amyloidosis, which is usually related to suppurative or chronic inflammatory diseases such as chronic rheumatoid arthritis or tuberculosis.

The amyloid protein is heterogenous and displays two main types. Amyloid L is seen in primary amyloidosis. This is secreted by plasma cells, and is related to light chains of immunoglobulins modified by macrophage ingestion. Usually it is linked to a serum protein called serum amyloid P to produce the final fibrillary protein which is deposited typically around blood vessels.

Amyloid A, found in secondary amyloidosis, is derived from an acute phase serum protein modified by macrophage ingestion which links with serum amyloid P to form the final fibrillary protein.

Amyloid is sometimes difficult to see in tissues with haematoxylin and eosin staining. It is relatively easily overlooked because it may resemble rather homogeneous acellular fibrous tissue. Congo red stain demonstrates amyloid with an orange colour (**16.17**). Amyloid also shows under polarised light as a birefringent apple-green colour (**16.18**). Fluorescent dyes such as thioflavine T can also be used.

METASTASES IN LYMPH NODES

Metastases in cervical lymph nodes often originate from a known primary carcinoma in the head and neck, usually from a visible lesion in the mouth or oropharynx. If, however, there is no obvious primary carcinoma, it may be necessary to perform an examination under general anaesthesia to look for a tumour, particularly in the nasopharynx. Sometimes, multiple blind biopsies from the nasopharynx or the posterior third of the tongue are required. If the metastasis is a poorly differentiated carcinoma and there is no obvious nasal, nasopharyngeal or other primary tumour, the nasopharynx is sometimes irradiated over a wide field on the basis that it is the most likely primary site despite the negative investigations.

Within the lymph node, the metastatic tumour may first appear either in the subcapsular sinus or in a more central location. With secondary squamous cell carcinoma in the neck it is important to report whether the tumour is still contained within the substance of the lymph node or whether it has spread through the capsule into the surrounding tissues. This worsens the prognosis and often changes the treatment required, for example, if there is extracapsular spread after neck block dissection, radical post-surgical radiotherapy is frequently undertaken.

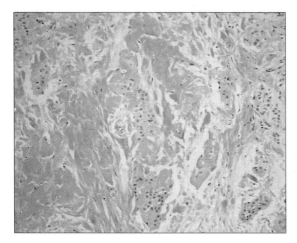

16.17 Amyloid. Congo red stain.

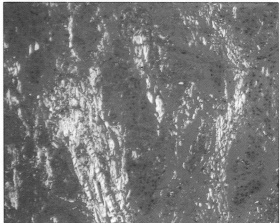

16.18 Amyloid. Congo red stain under polarised light.

INDEX